DR. DAVID JAMES WOOD
(1865-1937)

Father of Ophthalmology and First Medical Specialist
in South Africa

A Biography by
DR. JANET HODGSON
Granddaughter

Dr. Janet Hodgson © 2014

For my family
and
for all those who care for our sight.

TABLE OF CONTENTS

FOREWORD:
Dr. Gideon du Plessis: Ophthalmologist, Pretoria Eye Institute   9

PREFACE   11

PART 1   Early Years
Chapter 1   Scottish Roots   15
Chapter 2   Upbringing in Earlston and Galashiels   17
Chapter 3   Medical Training: Edinburgh and Moorfields   21

PART 2   Settling in South Africa
Chapter 4   From Ship's Doctor to Ophthalmologist   26
Chapter 5   Home Life at 'Gledsmuir', Plumstead   29
Chapter 6   Cars, Trains and Hansom Cabs   34
Chapter 7   Bottled Eyes and Brains   41
Chapter 8   Tinus de Jongh, Medical Artist   46

PART 3   Constance Clara Wood
Chapter 9   Family and Farming   50
Chapter 10   Suffragist and Town Councillor   54
Chapter 11   Jersey Cows, Ghosts, and the *Gita*   58

PART 4   'A Scientific Saint'
Chapter 12   Eye Doctor To All   64
Chapter 13   Surgeon, Teacher and Clinician   68
Chapter 14   Blind Lepers on Robben Island   73
Chapter 15   Vaccines, District Surgeons and Dentistry   77
Chapter 16   A Granddaughter's Treasure Hunt   81

PART 5   **'A Master of His Subject'**

Chapter 17   Founding an Ophthalmological Society   88
Chapter 18   Research and Writing in South Africa   92
Chapter 19   Dr. C. F. Louis Leipoldt, Editor and Colleague   97
Chapter 20   'The Blindness of John Milton'   101
Chapter 21   Celebrated Beyond South African Shores   107

PART 6   **'A Man's Best Monument'**   113

EPILOGUE
Dr. William Rowland: Past President of the World Blind Union, and Honorary Life President of both Disabled People South Africa and the S.A. National Council for the Blind.   117

Endnotes   119

Sources   135

Bibliography   138

Appendix 1: The Children of David James and Constance Clara Wood   141

Appendix 2: Ophthalmic Notes, Addresses and Articles in South Africa by Dr. D.J. Wood   141

Appendix 3:   Papers in the *British Journal of Ophthalmology* by D.J. Wood.   143

Appendix 4: The D.J. Wood Memorial Lectures   144

Appendix 5: Paintings of the Retina by Tinus de Jongh and Dr. D.J. Wood in the Department of Opthalmology, Groote Schuur Hospital, Cape Town.   145

Acknowledgements   147

Publications   150

List of Photographs: Julie Hodgson   150

Abbreviations

BJO – British Journal of Ophthalmology

BMA – British Medical Association

CGH – Cape of Good Hope (Western) Branch of the BMA

JMASA – Journal of the Medical Association of S.A. (B.M.A.)

OSSA – Ophthalmological Society of South Africa

SAMC – South African Medical Council

SAMJ – South African Medical Journal/S.A. Tydskrif vir Geneeskunde

SAMR – South African Medical Record

FOREWORD
Dr. Gideon du Plessis,
Ophthalmologist, Pretoria Eye Institute

It is a great privilege to write a foreword to the long awaited publication of Dr. Janet Hodgson on the life of Dr. David James Wood.

The Ophthalmological Society of South Africa decided to name its most prestigious lecture after D.J. Wood, the first ophthalmologist and first medical specialist in South Africa. Since then D.J. Wood has become familiar to every OSSA member through the D.J. Wood memorial lectures at their Congresses. For many years we only had scanty anecdotal information about the man himself, and only one photo that we saw annually at the lecture. If one, however, starts exploring the life of D.J. Wood, a character is revealed who has many remarkably different facets. These previously unknown aspects of his life and work are still relevant to any ophthalmologist today.

I endeavoured to open a small window of information about D.J. Wood through my personal research and discussions with some of his family - Mr. Geoff Montgomery and Mrs. Janet Sutherland - on the occasion of the D. J. Wood memorial lecture I presented in 2010. A man of high ethical values, Dr. D. J. Wood was dedicated to ophthalmology and promoted it among the medical fraternity of his time. He was much respected and well-loved by both his peers and his patients, locally and internationally. Always eager to introduce new thoughts and treatment modalities in the interest of his patients, his personal interests came second.

With the publication of Dr. Hodgson's book, for the first time we have a comprehensive history and full view of the life of Dr. D.J. Wood. It is indeed a singular milestone for Dr. Hodgson and for the Ophthalmological Society alike. She has created a record for posterity and a revelation to us in understanding more about the man. I believe that her book will confirm our perceptions of Dr. Wood and expand our knowledge and appreciation of him as a person and a medical practitioner. I want to congratulate Dr. Hodgson on the publication of this book. Thank you for the effort of collecting, editing and writing up the material. Thank you for your perseverance. We know that all this was done under difficult personal circumstances.

I am sure that this book will enlighten the discerning mind on the knowledge and understanding of Dr. D. J. Wood and his legacy, and that in future he will no longer be remembered merely as the name of a lecture.

I hope that every South African ophthalmologist as well as the general public will read the book and that it will be an edifying experience similar to the way I experienced it.

✧

PREFACE

My paternal grandfather, Dr. David James Wood, M.B., C.M., (Edinburgh), came to the Cape towards the end of 1893 and has the distinction of being the first full-time ophthalmologist in the country. He was also the very first specialist in medicine in South Africa.

The Ophthalmological Society of South Africa defines ophthalmology as 'the branch of medicine, which deals with the diseases and symptoms of the visual pathways, including the eye, brain and areas surrounding the eye'. (1) The annual D.J. Wood Memorial Lecture at the OSSA congresses have kept my grandfather's memory alive as the father of ophthalmology in South Africa but, as Dr. du Plessis says, up to now surprisingly little has been known about the all-encompassing nature of his life and work, a true Renaissance man. Who was Dr. D.J. Wood and why should he be so honoured?

In this biography I have scoured every possible source to record as much as I can about my grandfather's family background, personal history, hobbies, writing, contribution to ophthalmology at home and abroad, and medical services to a wide spectrum of society, many being free of charge. He always signed himself as D.J.W. on the corners of his drawings and paintings, and used his initials in correspondence and articles. In Britain there is a medical tradition whereby colleagues refer to each other by their initials. Many close associates knew him as D.J.W. and it is the name I will use to tell his story. It is a fascinating tale, a voyage of discovery, which has allowed me to make an amazing variety of new friends and opened windows on a totally new world.

Around 1935, D.J.W. wrote a ten page 'Retrospect - for my children, and those who will come after them', where he traces fragments of his Scottish ancestry. He much regretted that he had not taken more interest in family history earlier on. By then he had been practising in Cape Town for more than forty years. He continued working in his private practice, as an eye surgeon at the New Somerset Hospital, as lecturer in ophthalmology in the University of Cape Town Medical School, as a committee member of various medical bodies, and in his research and writing, until the last days of his life. He died from heart failure on 18th March 1937, aged seventy-one.

My grandmother, Constance Clara Wood (nee Cooke), was a formidable woman, very independent for her time, and of equal interest. After leaving England for South Africa in 1893, she married my grandfather two years later and soon carved out her own career. As a suffragist, she was a founding member of the women only Alexandra Club in Cape Town, treasurer of the Women's Unionist Society, and the first woman town councillor in Wynberg, in 1921. As a farmer in Plumstead, she was actively involved in running a large poultry concern and a dairy, where she bred pedigreed Jersey cattle. In 1926, she was a founding member of the Western Province Jersey Cattle Club and the only woman on the committee. As a mother, she brought up six children, three boys and three girls. She died in 1943 and is buried with my grandfather in Plumstead Cemetery.

Unfortunately, my grandfather was extremely modest about his own career. He ended his short 'Retrospect' with the words: 'To some other of you I leave the rest of the story'. This I have now tried to piece together with considerable difficulty. In his Retrospect, D.J.W. provides brief information about his early years, school and university education, medical training in Scotland and at the Moorfields Eye Hospital in London, and the start of his practice in Cape Town. My grandmother left no record of her life whatsoever so that this memorial to these two remarkable people has had to rely on oral family history to fill in many of the gaps.

The main sources of information regarding the family have been tape-recorded interviews I made with my father, Harry, and his younger brother, Donald, when they were in their late eighties. In addition, Geoff Montgomery, son of D.J.W.'s oldest daughter, Madge, provided me with a wealth of reminiscences about our grandparents. Now in his eighties, Geoff is the senior member of the family. As a young lad he was a regular visitor to the Wood family home and knew them well. Harry was born in 1904, Donald in 1912, and Geoff in 1928. All three were blessed with amazing memories and what has been impressive is the consistency of their anecdotes. Their recollections have dovetailed in essential details, while their stories were enriched by their personal experiences and particular take on events. My twin brother, James, who lives in Western Australia, is now the oldest surviving member of the Wood dynasty. We have two younger Wood cousins in New Zealand, Donald's sons.

Other material concerning my grandparents' lives has been gathered from a variety of sources. These include a small collection of family papers, reminiscences of people who knew D.J.W. including his patients, informative obituaries, forty-eight of his research papers of varying length (including addresses given at conferences and medical association meetings), and historical data relating to the medical world. I have also drawn on tantalisingly slight references to the role my grandmother played in Cape Town society and the context in which she functioned. In some instances I have had to use Internet sources knowing that they are not always reliable.

What started out as an article about my grandparents has grown into a book. They were both such amazing characters, and their paths crossed with interesting people like Sir Herbert Baker, Sir Lionel and Lady Phillips, Sir Murray Bisset, Sir Alfred Hennessy, Tinus de Jongh (to whom D.J.W. gave a start as a struggling artist), and the medical fraternity, including Dr. C. Louis Leipoldt.

Leipoldt was a medical colleague at the New Somerset Hospital and fellow lecturer at the start of the University of Cape Town Medical School. He also edited the *South African Medical Journal (SAMJ)* and was the first organising secretary of the South African Medical Association from the 1920s on. This was in addition to being a poet and writer in Afrikaans and English, playwright, botanist, and gourmet chef. D.J.W. was a valued contributor to his journal and, despite differences in age and political opinions, they became close friends. Leipoldt wrote an affectionate tribute to D.J.W. after his death.

This book is not a scientific treatise about my grandfather's contribution to ophthalmology. I leave that to the experts. Only they can do justice to his pioneering spirit and the visionary nature of his research. There is much of historic interest in his extensive writing as listed in the Appendices. His usage of the medical terminology of his time has been retained throughout for historical reasons, although much has been updated since then. These articles will be deposited in the Department of Opthalmology at Groote Schuur for research purposes. Even so they are not a complete collection.

What I have tried to do is to bring my grandparents to life as real people. Having ventured into the foreign field of ophthalmology, I apologise for any errors. I take courage from a story told me by Professor A.C. (Kay) de Villiers, former Head of the Department of Neurosurgery at UCT, although the application of the story is somewhat different in my case:

At the beginning of Neurosurgery in Britain, as elsewhere in the world, the physicians tried to determine the site of a cerebral tumour by means of clinical symptoms and signs as there were no investigations to assist them. The neurosurgeon, if he had the courage, had to operate on these, at times, flimsy fragments of evidence.

It is told of Victor (later Sir) Horsley that he operated at Queen's Square on the basis of such clinical localisation with the physician concerned watching from the gallery. Horsley opened the skull and found no tumour. In despair he threw up his hands and exclaimed: 'I am giving up neurosurgery!' The physician's response was: 'Don't give it up Victor, just take it up.' (2)

Although my Ph.D. is in Religious Studies (UCT 1985), I do have some scientific background with a research degree in Agriculture (cum laude) from Stellenbosch University (1957). In writing this book I realise that I am often working with 'flimsy fragments of evidence', open to misrepresentation, but take courage from friends and advisers.

I was born in January 1936, just over a year before my grandfather died, so I have no memory of him except through photographs. I owe him a debt of gratitude, however, as he put me in spectacles before I was a year old to straighten a squint, but I was still left with a 'lazy' (amblyopic) eye. Over the years my spectacles continued to be those round, owl-like ones with temples that curled behind my ears. Professor Tony Murray has some on display in glass cases in the ophthalmology museum at Groote Schuur Hospital. (3) I now rank with the museum pieces. After D.J.W.'s death, Dr. Leonard Townsend took over his practice in Church Square. The desk, cupboards and book shelves lining the walls were all made by my grandfather. I have vivid memories of regular visits to those dark rooms to have my eyes tested and spectacles changed.

Since I turned sixty I have had the gradual progression of Age-related Macular Degeneration (AMD). Happily the term Senile MD has been dropped. I have written a separate story on *Living With Low Vision*, which has been published on the Internet and as a booklet. Here, I have tried to use my own experience to share ideas on how to live as full a life as possible. I have also provided information on some of the available resources such as visual aids, audio devices, exercises, and support groups. The prevalence of AMD is surprisingly widespread among older people, often unacknowledged or ignored, so that they do not get the correct help and advice. Above all else is the need to be positive and face the problem squarely, to overcome the fear of losing one's sight and with it one's independence. Emotional and social concerns are almost as great as are the medical aspects of the disease.

✧

PART 1: EARLY YEARS
Chapter 1
Scottish Roots

David James Wood begins his 'Retrospect' by observing that neither nobility nor remarkable greatness appears in his family tree until one goes so far back that the records are doubtful. (1) Even so, he identifies those ancestors who, according to family tradition, made their mark in history. On his father's side they included Sir Andrew Wood, Admiral of the Scottish fleet in the time of James III. On his maternal side there was Sir William de Landale, who followed William the Conqueror from Normandy and was the most aristocratic of his forebears.

More immediate paternal relations, whom D.J.W. remembered meeting, included clergymen, schoolmasters, and a wine merchant in London. Some of their portraits and those of their wives hung in his home at 'Gledsmuir' at the Cape. One painting of his parents was so awful that his mother had burnt it. He treasured the pieces of furniture such as a number of presentation clocks and a sideboard, which he brought with him from Scotland.

Family information was hard to come by even in his day. Most records outside the nobility were lodged in the Session records of the Scottish Churches, and were either lost or destroyed. But D.J.W. believed that his father came from good yeoman stock, hard working artisans and farmers in the Lowlands of the Scottish Border. His great-great grandfather, George Shillinglaw, was 'a contractor' living near Melrose. One son, Joseph, did much of the woodwork at Abbotsford, the home of Sir Walter Scott on the River Tweed. Joseph made and carved the desk, preserved in Scott's library, at which he wrote his novels. Another son, D.J.W.'s great grandfather (1775-1836), was a nurseryman and supplied most of the trees on the Abbotsford Estate. One plantation was known as 'Shillinglaw's Plantin'. In the 1990s, Scott's two elderly granddaughters were much intrigued to learn of this information when we met them in the rose garden on a visit to Abbotsford.

D.J.W.'s relations on both sides had large families. His Shillinglaw grandmother, Helen, was one of ten children. In 1789 she married James Wood, proprietor of the gas works at Earlston (also spelt Earlstoun), a small market town in the county of Berwickshire on the Borders, 40 km from Edinburgh. Helen had twelve children. D.J.W.'s father, James (1831-1896), was the eighth in his family. The gas works were inherited by his eldest brother, George. Since it was difficult to find work for younger sons, James was apprenticed to John Cochrane who had the principal drapery in Galashiels, 20 km west of Earlston.

Galashiels is on the Gala Water River. With its twenty-two mills it was then a prosperous commercial centre famous for its high-quality textiles. D.J.W. noted that Gala tweed was 'synonymous with an all wool cloth where neither shoddy nor cotton were allowed to adulterate it'. Cochrane was a good friend to James and made no objections when he started his own establishment in the town. By this time he had married Christina (also known as Christiana) Smith Walker (1825-1905), Smith being her grandmother's name. She continued to live in her father's house in Earlston until his death, while James commuted weekly to Galashiels. It was Christina who recorded her side of the family's history in her many handwritten notebooks, some of which are in our possession.

Christina came from a long line of linen weavers going back to David Walker, a master weaver in Cupar Fife in the early 18th century. Her father, also David Walker, was supposed to take up the trade of cabinet-maker. However, he was academically bright and his schoolmaster persuaded Walker senior to send him to Edinburgh to train for the ministry in the Church of Scotland. David started his further education in 1800 but as this involved considerable expense, he earned extra money as a private tutor. During one vacation he had only just started work with a family in the countryside when they detected his Berwickshire burr. He was promptly dispatched with a five-pound note as compensation. This he used to buy a handsome watch. He eventually lost the burr but not the watch and it became a family heirloom.

Later on, David was teaching in a parish school near Coldingham. Young, good looking, intelligent and a diligent churchgoer, he was frequently invited to dine at the manse. There he met Margaret Landell, second daughter of the minister, and the young couple fell in love. They knew that their parents would never agree to a marriage until David had completed his nine years of training for the ministry and had set up a respectable home. Consequently, they ran away to Edinburgh to be married. This scandalous behaviour caused their parents much grief.

As marriage was then a bar to preferment in the church, David took up teaching as a profession. Having received a first class Scottish education, he was not only proficient in English, Latin, Greek and Mathematics, but also Hebrew and French, with some German and Italian as well. He taught in a number of parish schools before a better position in Earlston became available. This was not without drama as the schoolmaster's post was keenly contested by highly qualified candidates. A formal examination was set up in the Earlston Court Room to put the final two contestants through a stiff selection process. Both managed to solve a difficult Mathematics problem but David won through with his ability to translate an obscure Greek passage. He remained at Earlston for the rest of his life.

Christina Smith Walker was the youngest of his four children, being born in Edinburgh on 13ᵗʰ September 1859. Her eldest brother, another James, was the only one in the family who ever made money. He had a business in London as an outfitter of men going abroad to India or for those joining the army. He supplied them with everything from clothing to weapons. David, the second son, was a doctor but died young from consumption. Harriet, the other daughter, married a lighterman working on the River Thames in London. His work involved transferring goods from a ship to a wharf or another ship in a flat-bottomed boat. They too had a large family but the eldest son eventually squandered the once thriving business.

Christina was given an excellent education including time spent in France to learn the language. Besides the notebooks documenting the Walker family history, she kept diaries recording her daily life, made lively observations on local history and natural phenomena, and researched the genealogies of neighbouring families. Her marble bust ended up in our double storey home in Retreat, standing on a plinth at the bottom of the stairs. Its ghostly whiteness with its tightly ordered coiffure and stern demeanour was a terrifying spectacle in the dark. Fortunately, it was eventually replaced by a grandfather clock.

Chapter 2
Upbringing in Earlston and Galashiels

David James Wood was born in the schoolhouse Hunt Pools, Earlston, on 4ᵗʰ July 1865. Earlston is on the River Leader in Lauderdale, a market town on the main road from Northumberland in north-east England to Edinburgh. As a small child D.J.W. remembered going for drives in a pony-chaise, shaped like a basket with seats facing towards each other and very low. By this time his grandfather was partly paralysed and the pony-chaise enabled him to get out and about for fresh air. D.J.W. also recalled being spilt out of a perambulator while still living at Earlston, and of being taken to the river bridge at weekends to wave to his father on his return home from Galashiels. He believed that he had inherited his small hands, ideal for delicate eye operations, from his mother and grandmother.

As a youngster, D.J.W. was awed by the big books with their battered old bindings in his grandfather Walker's school library. There were shelves on Mathematics (including the 11ᵗʰ and 12ᵗʰ books of Euclid), and piles of Greek and Latin works. Sadly, they were all thrown away when the family moved to Galashiels after his grandfather's death. As D.J.W. later observed: 'Neither the men nor such books can

EXTRACT OF AN ENTRY IN A REGISTER OF **BIRTHS**,
of 17° and 18° Victoriæ,
kept in the undermentioned PARISH OR DISTRICT, in terms
Cap. 80, § § 56 & 58.

No.	Name and Surname.	When and Where Born.	Sex.	Name, Surname, and Rank or Profession of Father. Name, and Maiden Surname of Mother. Date and Place of Marriage.	Signature and Qualification of Informant, and Residence, if out of the House in which the Birth occurred.	When and Where Registered, and Signature of Registrar.
42	David James Wood. Vaccinated etc. Certificat dated 10th Sep 1865 R.S. Ray?	1865 July Fourth 2h 40m. P.M. Earlston	M	James Wood Draper Christina Wood m.s. Smith Walker 1859 Sept 15th at Edinburgh	(Signed) James Wood Father	1865 July 26th at Earlston (Signed) Robt Smith Registrar

Extracted from the Register Book of Births, for the _Parish_ of _Earlston_, in the _County_ of _Berwick_, this _6th_ day of _November_ _1900_   _Robt Smith_ Registrar.

David James Wood's Birth Certificate (2)

today be found save in the highest class schools, whereas he taught in a village of some 1000 people.'

His youngest sister, Eleanor, died when she was three. His older sister, Harriet Margaret, was a brilliant student, furthering her studies at Heidelberg University. However, she had a quick temper and maybe that is why she never married. As a schoolmistress her fiery disposition was problematic with her pupils. She visited the Wood family twice in South Africa and they found her extremely difficult. According to Donald, the youngest of my father's five siblings, my grandmother, Constance, could not stand her sister-in-law and called her 'a bitch'. As a dedicated suffragist Harriet is supposed to have gone up in a balloon over the Cape Peninsula in order to distribute pamphlets.

When my grandparents' eldest daughter was born, Aunt Harriet was somewhat miffed that she was christened Marjorie Constance Christina (known as Madge) and not named after her. With my father's arrival more than four years later, he was called Harry to placate the old lady and keep her quiet.

D.J.W.'s father, James Wood, hated his draper's business. He was cramped in a dark shop, selling things he loathed, and with few breaks from one year to the next. However, he was determined to give his children the best education he could and his self-sacrifice allowed them to spend a month each summer at the seaside. Coldingham was their favourite place, they being close friends with the 'Manse people' who had succeeded the Landells. In later life, James Wood took up the business of wool buying and was more successful in this trade with less arduous hours.

In his reminiscences, D.J.W. maintained that his mother undoubtedly married beneath her in a pecuniary sense. None the less, his parents were a devoted couple sharing 'the same love of antiquities and the same devotion to their church, and nation'. His father collected old books, his special interest being the days of 'the Covenanters'. Some volumes in his library, like an early 'Ben Johnson', were valuable. Both Woods were keen members of the Berwickshire Naturalist's Club, a forerunner of many such societies in Britain devoted to saving places of historic interest from ruin. Christina wrote numerous articles for the club based on research in old records. These were published in local newspapers and journals. James was also an elder in his church and superintendent of the Sunday School. His son relates that 'he never questioned any of the church's teachings, nor made any enemies'. Christina was a devout churchgoer, too, and would reflect on the weekly Bible readings and sermons in her diaries. Both of them were fervent members of the Temperance Movement. James Wood died in 1896 and Christina in 1904, they being buried alongside other family members in the Earlston cemetery.

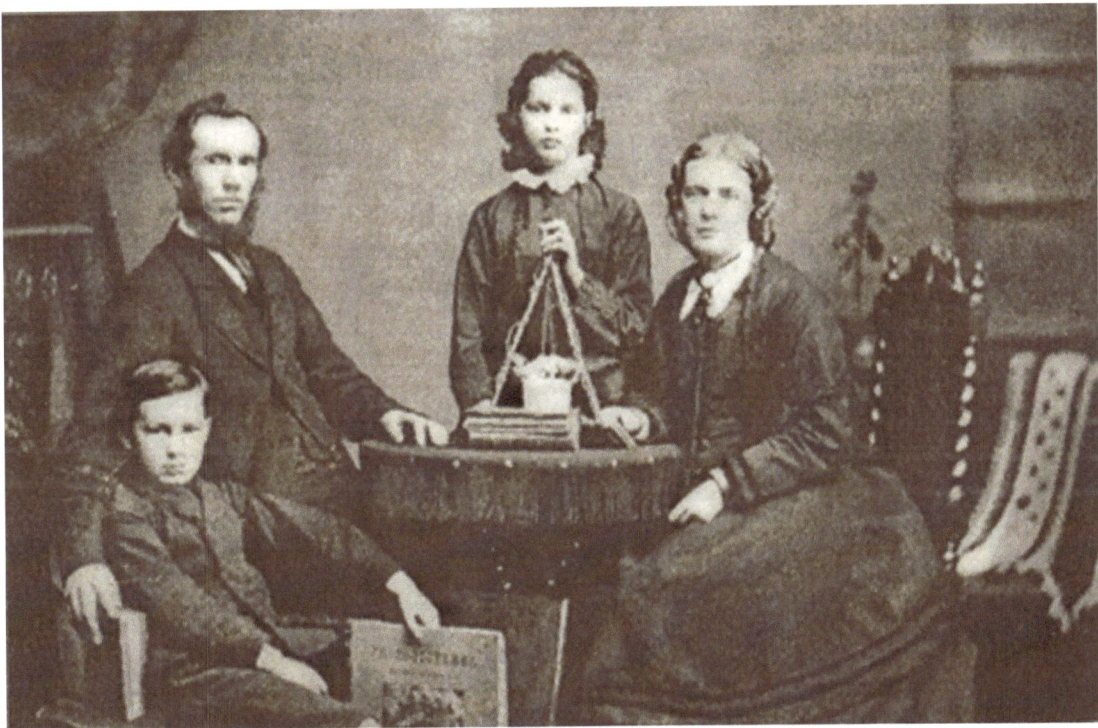

Wood Family, Earlston (3)

Harriet had a memorial window to her parents placed in St. Paul's Church, Galashiels, in 1906. The inscription reads: 'Giving thanks for the lives of James and Christina Wood, and so they came unto their desired haven.' The window was 'dedicated by their children' but D.J.W. only ever saw a photograph. We tracked it down on a visit to the church. We also visited the numerous family graves in Earlston cemetery, braving the pouring rain. It was a strange experience to see the engravings of Janet and James Wood, the names of myself and my twin brother, on many headstones. My grandfather set great store by the fact that over several generations on both sides of his family, 'there were none other than respectable citizens, many earning the love and esteem of all who knew them'.

After they moved to Galashiels, D.J.W.'s was for many years taught at home by his well-educated mother, from whom he learnt much. When he was twelve he was sent to Galashiels Academy. This was the first time he had mixed with boys of his own age, but he found them 'mostly rather inferior in knowledge'. Both in Galashiels, and at his next school, Highfield in Melrose, he had the bad luck of being placed in a class with boys much older than himself, probably because of his advanced education. He had to put up with a good deal of roughness, which, with his slight build, he was not able to return. Most of the boys were farmers' sons, some from a fair distance away. D.J.W. thought them rather dull and much regretted that he had made far less progress at school than could have been expected.

From Melrose he went on to the Royal High School in Edinburgh, where 'the late King Edward had been a pupil for some two years, long before my time'. The school had been founded in 1128 and was one of the oldest in the world. Run by the Scottish Church, it had initially provided a Latin education for the sons of landed and burgess families, many of them going on to serve the Church. (1) By the late 19th century its Public School education offered Latin, Greek, French, German, English, History, Geography, Mathematics and Science. Fencing, military drill and gymnastics were also part of the curriculum. Over the years the school occupied a number of different sites. During D.J.W.'s time it was located in the Regent Road building on Calton Hill. Boarders lived in 'The House' in Royal Terrace. The school uniform was a formal black and white. Old boys included the Scottish poets and writers, Robert Fergusson and Walter Scott, and Alexander Graham Bell, eminent scientist, engineer and inventor of the first telephone. (2)

Two of D.J.W.'s school friends from Galashiels, James Somerville and William Rutherford, accompanied him to Edinburgh. Rutherford went through the medical course with him, too, and remained a trusted friend of the family. The teaching staff at the Royal School was said to be first class but some masters struggled to control their students. One very eminent man, a fine classical scholar, was seen going into the 'Thistle' tavern. After that he was pretty much at the mercy of the young devils who knew about his fall from grace.

Because of D.J.W.'s changes of school and indifferent teaching, he was behind in some subjects, especially the Classics. He made up for it, however, in French and German. At the end of his second year he was sixth in class and 'Dux' of the school in French, but still way down in the Classics. He stayed on another year but by then the school had been handed over by the City Council to a School Board and a new principal, Dr. Marshall, had been appointed. There was an immediate drop in the institution's prestige and it took some time to recover. After he left D.J.W. felt that royalty would no longer have favoured the Royal High.

His next academic hurdle was to pass the Edinburgh University entrance examination. He did well enough 'except for one mortification'. Because of his earlier difficulties with schooling he failed Arithmetic. Even so he had only one 'bare pass'. Otherwise he achieved several 'Bs' and some 'BBs' (*bene*). At the second go he managed to scrape through Arithmetic with Logic and Greek, but Mathematics remained a weakness in his further studies.

Chapter 3
Medical Training: Edinburgh and Moorfields

At Edinburgh University, D.J.W. says that he worked hard at the subjects he liked; but only put in enough effort with the less favoured ones to get passes. (1) He gained class medals in Chemistry, Medicine and Ophthalmology, and also took the certificate in mental diseases, but was dissuaded from going in for this speciality. (My brother has his large brass medal in Ophthalmology.) On 1st August 1888, he graduated with the degree of Bachelor of Medicine and Master of Surgery. He hoped to become a house physician, but did not know that the usual examination for these posts in the infirmary had been abolished. This meant that he did not apply to his chief, Professor Greenfield, until too late. Fortunately, there was a second option and he was taken on by Dr. Douglas Moray Cooper Lamb Argyll Robertson as a house surgeon in the eye wards at Edinburgh Hospital. The only problem was that this post was not a residential appointment leaving him to struggle financially.

Argyll Robertson was one of the first surgeons to specialise in the field of ophthalmology and he taught at Edinburgh University from 1883 to 1897. Tradition has it that he fought a duel to win the hand of his wife, possibly the last fought in Britain if it actually took place. He is best remembered for the 'Argyll Robertson Pupil or Syndrome' of the eye. This was a common symptom of neurosyphilis and other diseases of the central nervous system. The syndrome is characterized by the pupils constricting or accommodating when the patient focuses on a near object, but they fail to constrict when exposed to bright light. They were originally known as 'prostitute's pupils' because of their association with tertiary syphilis; and 'because of the convenient mnemonic that, like a prostitute, they "accommodate but do not react"'. (2)

Argyll Robertson's other claim to fame was as a golfer, winning the gold medal of the Royal and Ancient Club of St. Andrew five times. D.J.W. said that he could never forget the high born courtesy of his mentor, nor the charm of his beautiful wife. Dr. Jospeh Bell, a physician with a special interest in forensic medicine, was one of his lecturers at Edinburgh. Arthur Conan Doyle was a fellow student. He became Bell's house surgeon and dedicated his portrayal of Sherlock Holmes to Bell together with Dr. Watson. James Barrie, author of *Peter Pan*, and Robert Louis Stevenson, author of *Treasure Island*, were other students at this time. (3) After the nine months needed to complete his housemanship at Edinburgh, D.J.W. was appointed clinical assistant at the Royal London Ophthalmological Hospital, Old Moorfields, in London.

'Moorfields' was the first specialist eye hospital, the oldest and largest in the world. It was opened on the Moorfields Common in 1805 as the London Dispensary for curing diseases of the Eye and Ear. Situated near the Moorgate, the Moorfields was one of the last pieces of open land available in London. The fields had had a chequered history, being used as a refugee encampment for impoverished and displaced people after the Great Fire in 1666. As the centuries progressed the fields provided space for occasional fairs, shows and auctions. This was a poor area, acquiring an unsavoury reputation for harbouring highwaymen and fugitives from the law, and for keeping brothels and encouraging the cruising of gay men. Its notoriety was exacerbated by violent rioting during 1780. Respectability arrived with the establishment of a high-class carpet manufactory on the land in the mid 18th century, making way for further developments. (4)

The founding of the Royal London Ophthalmological Hospital was apparently motivated by an epidemic of trachoma, a form of potentially blinding conjunctivitis. British troops had brought back the eye disease on returning to England after the Napoleonic wars in Egypt. (5) An increasing growth in the number of patients seeking treatment led to the hospital having to be moved to larger sites, in 1822 and again in 1899, while retaining its original name. During D.J.W.'s time it was still functioning as a charity. On admission a patient would be given a card that read: 'This letter was granted to the applicant being poor. Its acceptance therefore by anyone not really poor constitutes an abuse of charity'. (6)

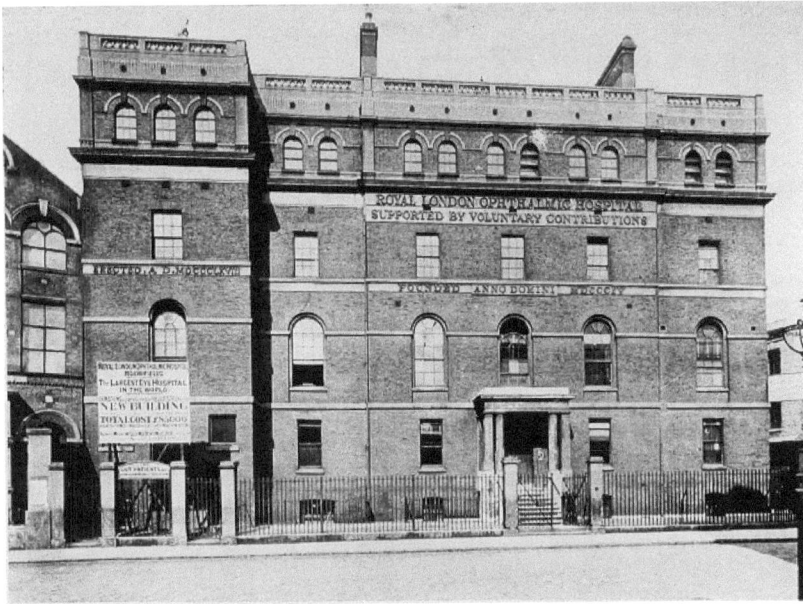

Moorfields Eye Hospital, London, 1875 (4)

At Moorfields D.J.W. worked under the leading consultants in ophthalmology of the day – Richard Marcus Gunn, a former student of Dr. Argyll Robertson (7), John Couper (8), Arthur Quarry Silcock (9) and Edward Nettleship (10). As pioneers in their fields, with wide medical and surgical expertise, they inspired his interest in research. This resulted in his spending two days a week with Silcock in the pathological laboratory at St. Mary's Hospital. At that stage there were no regular classes, 'you just soaked in the work and learned what your chiefs suggested'. During D.J.W.'s time at Moorfields, from 1889 to 1891, he found Gunn and Nettleship to be the most outstanding teachers. When Gunn became senior surgeon at the hospital in 1907, he followed Vienna's example in introducing a systematic teaching of eye disease. Nettleship, in turn, was highly regarded as a teacher of post-graduate studies in addition to his research on hereditary eye diseases. He is reported to have 'set exacting standards of clinical observation and documentation. He did not suffer fools gladly, but his enthusiasm and personality attracted the best students'. (11) D.J.W's youngest son was given the name Donald Nettleship Walker Wood.

As Dr. Gideon du Plessis notes, the involvement of Drs. John Couper and A. Stanford Morton in developing the modern ophthalmoscope of Helmholtz (1865), and their collaboration with Dr. Jackson in Colorado in developing the retinoscope, allowed D.J.W. to be part of the first group of ophthalmologists to more accurately determine refraction. But retinal surgery did not exist and the medicines available were minimal. There were no antibiotics and they had to rely on 'bismuth, boric acid, silver nitrate, cadmium, copper acetate, iodine, mercury citrine ointment and much more for almost any indication'. (12)

In November 1889, D.J.W. published a small *Handbook on Human Anatomy*, *Physiology and Hygiene* (London: Ruddiman Johnston & Co. Ltd.). He used this as a teaching aid in conjunction with the projection of Figures, at least some of which were drawn by himself. The Handbook to Sheet IV, in the Wood Papers and signed by the author, deals with 'Intoxicants and Narcotics. Drainage and Ventilation, Etc.' Each section is provided with a corresponding couple of Figures, numbered from I to XXXV, although the original illustrations have been lost. The sections on Alcohol, Water, Air and Ventilation have a series of simple experiments added to them to illustrate his presentation.

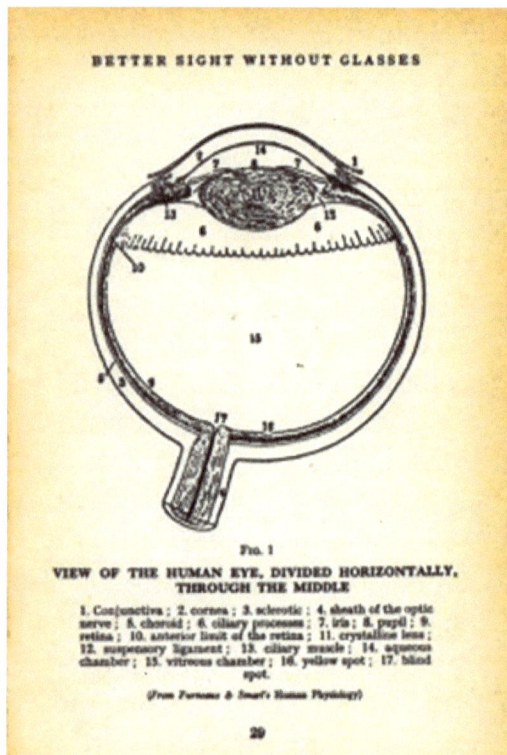

View of the Human Eye –
Harry Benjamin (1929) (5)

Although D.J.W. begins by describing the properties of alcohol, and its value in preserving animal structures and in producing methylated spirits, his strong temperance upbringing seems to have inspired his concern about the damaging effect it had on the body. He goes into some detail in discussing the diseases, which habitual indulgence of alcohol inflict on major organs like the liver, kidneys, brain, lungs, stomach and heart: 'This gives rise to fatty degeneration and formation of fibrous connective tissue. It greatly lessens muscular power and diminishes or suspends the action of the whole nervous system, beginning with the highest faculties.' His simple experiments with alcohol are used to show how it is lighter than water: how it produces heat in water: and how coagulation takes place when an egg white is poured into it, which can then be dissolved by the speedy addition of water. He concludes that, 'the habit of alcohol drinking is very easily induced but most difficult to check'. (p.4) Further on he gives a summary of 'The Effects of Alcohol on the Various Organs from Dr. Parkes "Practical Hygiene"'. (pp.14-17)

He also devotes a few pages to the harmful effects of nicotine in smoking tobacco, because this poisonous alkaloid is passed with the smoke into the system: 'In non-fatal doses it causes great sickness, prostration, and failure of the heart, symptoms which are well seen when tobacco is used for the first time in smoking'. In a pipe some nicotine is condensed in the stem, and does not get inhaled, while in cigarettes and cigars all is inhaled. However, the cigar is preferred to the pipe, as in a cigar most of the nicotine is changed into less active substances and is not so harmful. Even so, 'over-indulgence in smoking causes irritation of the throat and dyspeptic symptoms; while a still more formidable result is a serious impairment of vision'. (pp.18-19) A man ahead of his time. D.J.W. concludes that tobacco must be looked on as a pure luxury, doing more harm than good.

The main part of the booklet is taken up with describing the functions of different parts of the body, starting with the salivary glands, tongue and stomach, and continuing with the intestines, liver, arteries, heart, brain, and kidneys. Each section refers to numbered Figures. These again feature in his final demonstration on the impurities found in water and air, which were thought to be the cause of many serious diseases such as typhoid, malaria, dysentery, cholera and scarlet fever. (pp.19-23) The Handbook ends with notes on the importance of good ventilation and sanitation in any residence. (pp.23-31) There is no doubt that during his training as an eye surgeon D.J.W. followed his illustrious teachers in having a broad interest in medicine as a whole, and this remained with him for the rest of his life.

After eighteen months at Moorfields, D.J.W. was appointed junior house surgeon. Eighteen months later he was promoted to the senior position. The eye hospital was at the end of Blomfield Street, opposite Broad Street Station, and he found it 'noisy and uncomfortable in all respects. Still with but one breakdown I managed to carry on'. The hospital work for a senior house surgeon was demanding and the pay poor. The juniors got 50 pounds a year and the seniors 75 pounds. D.J.W. struggled to make ends meet. By the time he had paid for clothes, and the means for getting about, there was little money left for other necessities.

At the end of a particularly strenuous year in which no sunshine was recorded for forty days during one spell of winter, he developed a chest complaint and felt completely 'knocked out'. He was advised to leave the British climate and took sail as a ship's doctor to Spain and Portugal. Although it was 'a horrid trip' he made the most of the fresh air and sunshine. With his time now up at the hospital, and no money to make a start on his own, he was at his wit's end as to what to do next. After some delay he was taken on by what became the Union Castle Mail Steamship Company as a ship's surgeon. In those days the weekly mail contract on these passenger ships was shared between the Union Line and the Castle Shipping Line. The mail boats sailed on alternate weeks, the voyage taking three weeks. They eventually amalgamated to form the Union-Castle Line.

✦

PART 2 : SETTLING IN SOUTH AFRICA

Chapter 4
From Ship's Doctor to Ophthalmologist

D.J.W.'s first post as ship's doctor was on the S.S. Methuen Castle, a vessel of 2600 tons in which he sailed to Cape Town. He recalls that the ship was 'an old tub, unseaworthy and filled with immigrants'. It had no electricity and no cold storage. Fortunately, there were few passengers. Prior to his next trip he was transferred to the Warwick Castle, which brought out the first large consignment of Jewish people to South Africa. On this second voyage he met his future wife, Constance Clara Cooke, who was on her way to take up a post as a teacher in Durban. Having become romantically attached to Constance, and with no promising prospects in Britain, he decided to emigrate to South Africa. She appears to have returned to England in the interim because they both sailed from Southampton on board the Scot on 28th October 1893. In those days detailed passenger lists were kept, they being published in the Cape Town newspapers together with a log of the ship's journey.

D.J.W. arrived in Cape Town with only forty pounds in his pocket and some letters of recommendation. These were from the senior surgeons and professors at Moorfields - Warren Tay (1), Marcus Gunn, John Couper, Edward Nettleship, John Tweedy (2) and William Lang (3). Before he left home his mother made copies of these testimonials in one of her many notebooks, thus saving them for posterity. All spoke of Dr. Wood as a pleasant colleague with an outstanding intellect; his competent and detailed knowledge of every branch of ophthalmology; his exceptionally wide practical experience as a surgeon; his energy and punctiliousness in carrying out his duties; and his tenacity of purpose. In true Victorian spirit he was also a gentleman, who would reflect credit on any institution with which he might be associated. The surgeons confidently asserted that Dr. Wood had a brilliant career ahead of him and much regretted that he had not chosen to remain at Moorfields.

On coming to Cape Town at the end of 1893, D.J.W. made the brave decision to set up practice as an ophthalmologist, registering under the Old Cape Register. This gave him the distinction of being the first true medical specialist in South Africa, the start of many firsts. Prior to this, doctors had been expected to be competent in every branch of medicine and surgery, although some had developed certain specialities. At this time, Dr. Fismer, a German physician, did some eye work in Cape Town in addition to his general practice, as did Dr. Manikus. Whereas D.J.W., and later Dr. Napier in Johannesburg and Dr. Symonds in Kimberley, confined themselves to ophthalmology.

Shortly after arriving D.J.W. received another twenty pounds from Moorfields and opened up consulting rooms in a house in St. George's Street, Cape Town. He notes that he only managed to survive and become self-supporting by avoiding all but the bare necessities of life and by using his waiting room to live and sleep in. This had to be made ready each morning before the arrival of his first patients. He told his friend and colleague, Dr. E. Barnard Fuller, who commenced practice with him in 1893 as a surgeon, that 'it was uphill work at first but he won through and he never deviated from the path of specialism he had adopted'. (4)

Constance was also staying in Cape Town and she helped to improve his primitive living conditions. At weekends they would go on long walks up the mountain. Her love of animals remained with her all her life, and after putting in a whole day of tramping they would invariably have to carry the first of her many dogs home. Once D.J.W.ood's income had increased sufficiently to support the two of them they married in St. George's Cathedral in 1895, the imposing centre of the Anglican Church in Cape Town.

The *South African Medical Journal (SAMJ)* of December that year records that on the occasion of Dr. D.J. Wood's marriage, 'a number of medical gentlemen in Cape Town and district presented him with a handsome wedding present'. (5) The present included a dessert service, fruit knives and forks, and 'a Corinthian column dining-room lamp'. The names of twenty-two doctors are given, one of them being Jane Waterston. (6) The report notes that the wedding gift was partly a personal tribute to Dr. Wood, and partly a tribute to the good services he had rendered, and was continuing to give, as a most energetic secretary to the Cape Town Branch of the British Medical Association.

The Woods set up home in a tiny house at the foot of Breda Street. Howard, the eldest of their six children, was born here in 1897. As D.J.W.'s practice prospered so they were able to build their own house, 'Edgehill', in Belle Ombre Road, Tamboerskloof. This is where Marjorie (Madge) and Harry (my father) were born in 1899 and 1904 respectively. They soon outgrew this dwelling, and they also found the neighbourhood 'not very pleasant'. Constance wished to live in style and so in 1905 they moved to a newly opened up area in Plumstead, in the southern suburbs, where they built their imposing family home, 'Gledsmuir'. Patsy (1907), Rosamund (1909) and Donald (1912) were born here. According to Donald, his arrival was a rather unwelcome surprise.

D.J.W. recalls that in those days he soon had all the work he could manage and that 'there was no racial feeling'. Strangely enough this reference was to the growing Jewish community in Cape Town. He charged a one-guinea fee for a consultation, and great was his excitement when his day's takings amounted to twenty pounds in golden sovereigns. This was a decent income for income tax was less than two shillings in the pound. By 1906 the Voter's Roll records that D.J.W. had moved his consulting rooms to 41 Parliament Street in Church Square, opposite the 'Groote Kerk' of the Dutch Reformed Church. The property was valued at two thousand pounds. This entitled him to three votes in the Third Municipal District of Cape Town.

In his Reminiscences, D.J.W. writes that these happy days lasted many years. Towards the end of his life, however, he became embittered by the fact that of the seven ophthalmic surgeons then practising in Cape Town, a number were of Jewish origin and they had succeeded in attracting 'their own people out of my hands'. He maintained that up to this time there had been more than enough work for all. Now he despaired because he had been forced 'to go back to his first trouble to get people to know that I existed, except now it is to get them to know that I still exist after forty and more years of work'. Indeed, his complaint was a reality. In the mid 1930s he submitted a notice to the *SAMJ* in which he emphatically denied that he had retired, and asserted that he was very definitely still practising and intended to do so for some time to come.

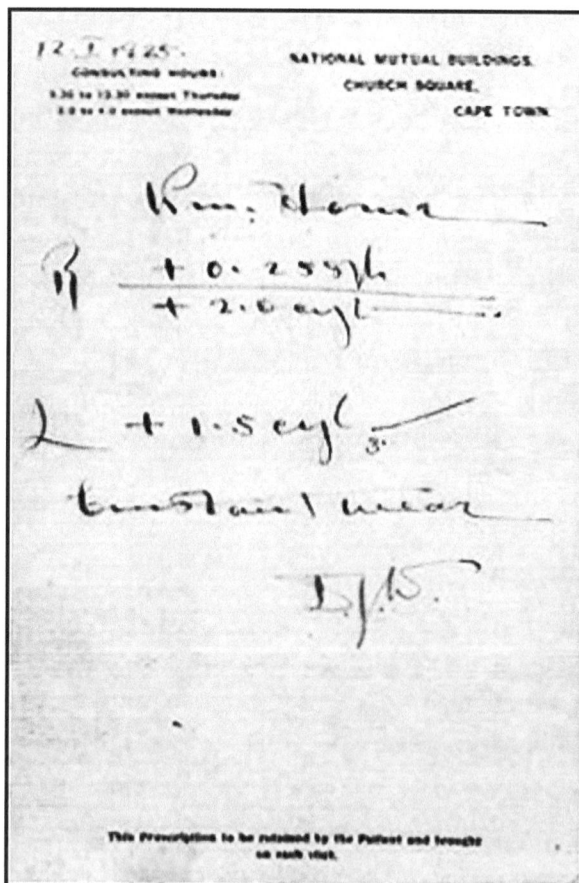

Prescription, 12.1.1925,
signed D.J.W. (6)

Although he might have felt resentful of the competition, his track record speaks of a much admired and valued specialist in his field whose pioneering work in ophthalmology was lauded by the medical fraternity both at home and abroad. Amongst his few papers is a letter dated May 1936 from a Mr. J. Foster F.R.C.S. in Leeds who had been consulted as to whether a South African eye patient should travel to England for further treatment. Having read D.J.W.'s report, Foster replied that, 'Mr. Wood, has among eye specialists, the reputation of being the best man in the South African Dominion, and his opinion can be taken as being as good as anybody's in Europe. I hesitate, always, to say that a case is hopeless, until I have had a chance of seeing it, and examining it; but quite frankly, on Wood's report, I do not think it worth while for this gentleman travelling to Europe for further opinions.'

Another wealthy woman went to England to consult an eye surgeon in Harley Street, only to be told by the great man: 'I don't know why you have come all this long way to see me when you have Wood in Cape Town.'

Chapter 5
Home Life at 'Gledsmuir', Plumstead

The Woods bought their land at Plumstead, on the western edge of the Cape Flats, from Colonel Southey. Originally, it had been the site of an old Dutch East India Company (VOC) camp. Then in the early 18th century it was granted to two Free Burghers as a farm. They called it 'Rust en Werk' (Rest and Work). This was part of the earliest wine growing area in the Cape stretching from below Wynberg, the wine being of decidedly poor quality. After the British Occupation, the farm was bought in 1828 by an Englishman, Henry Batt. He was a prosperous wine merchant and seller of dry goods to the navy. Batt renamed it Plumstead after his former home in London. As plots of land were sold off a pretty little village, also called Plumstead, sprang up along both sides of the wagon-road to Simonstown. The dusty track running through the village was lined with pine trees on the one side and a deep donga on the other.

Plumstead gradually expanded as tradesmen set up small businesses catering for the needs of the local farming community. In addition to a growing Muslim social group, these included emancipated slaves and free blacks. After Batt died in 1833, the property was subdivided and bought by a consortium of three men, one of whom was Southey. (1)

Lieutenant-Colonel Richard Southey was the son of Sir Richard Southey, a high-ranking civil servant at the Cape who had served with distinction in a number of frontier wars. In 1896, Colonel Southey bought the entire Plumstead property to farm with cattle. He named his estate 'Southfields'. The Wood boys remembered his cows being taken down to the vlei, now part of the Royal Cape Golf Club, to be watered morning and evening. Colonel Southey was known to walk around his land with the seeds of pine trees in his pocket. He would drop one seed at a time into a hole made by his walking stick, hence all the pine trees that flourished in Plumstead.

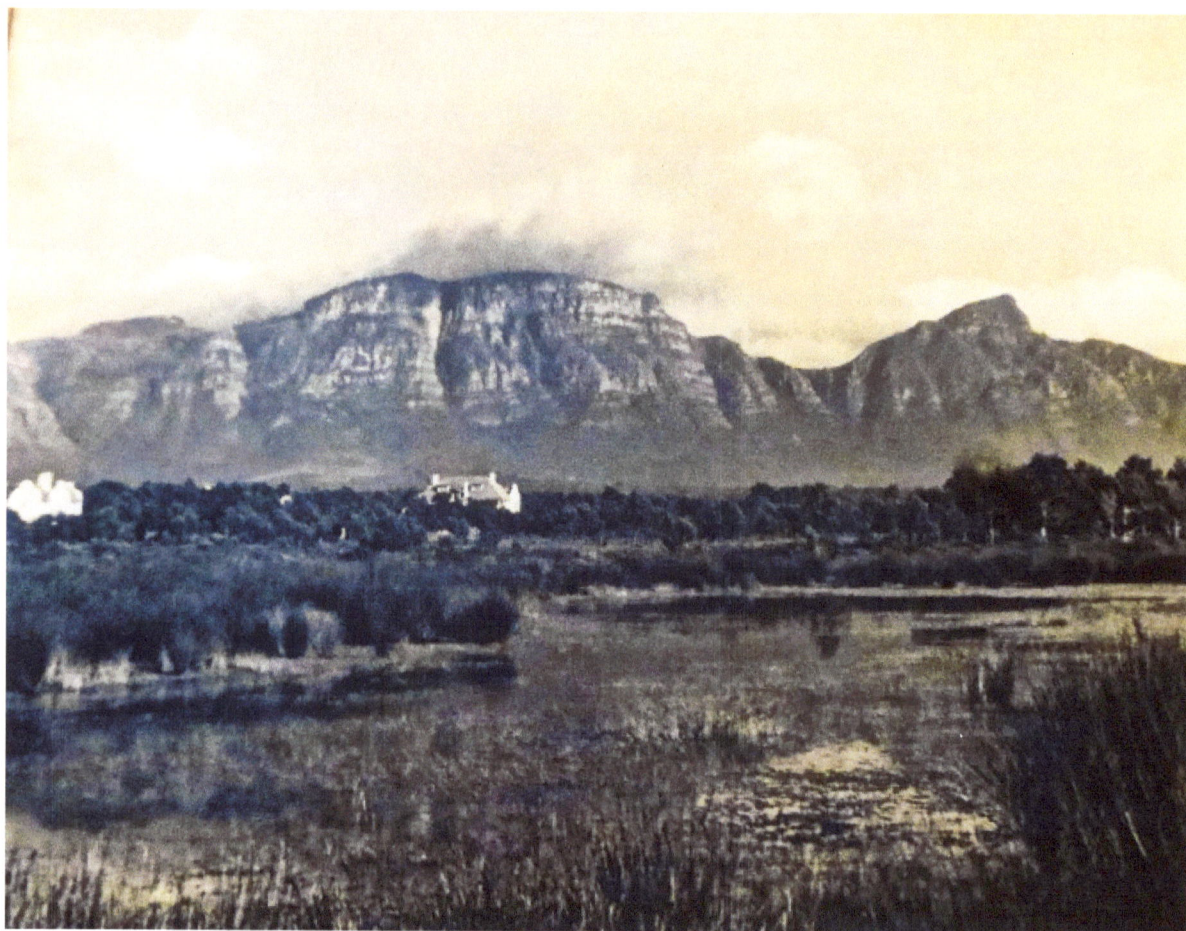

Photograph of 'Gledsmuir' from the Vlei by D.J.W. in the early 1910s
(Murray Bisset's house to the left). (7)

Besides his farming activities, he was Commander of Volunteers throughout the country, having previously served in the British Army. (2)

The Woods bought about four acres of ground from him on Southfield Road, plot number 6, extending as far as Prince George Drive. One of the neighbouring landowners were the Bissets, their property being closer to the railway line. Murray Bisset, whose father had been Mayor of Wynberg, had been admitted to the Cape Bar in 1899 and had a flourishing law practice. He was also a keen cricketer and as wicket keeper-batsman he had captained the South African cricket team against a visiting English side in 1897. Aged twenty-two, he was the youngest ever captain in Test cricket and this record was not broken for sixty years. He also captained the South African side when it toured England in 1901. In 1914, he was elected to the House of Assembly, representing the South African Party for South Peninsula. His political interests may well have influenced my grandmother to become involved in both municipal and party politics. In 1924, Bisset moved to Southern Rhodesia where he became Chief Justice and served twice as Acting-Governor during the Governor's absence, in 1928 and 1931. He was knighted in 1928. (3)

Other neighbours included Judge Fitzpatrick, whose son, Percy, wrote *Jock of the Bushveld*, and the Balls of Mrs Ball's chutney fame. Olive Schreiner, author of *Story of an African Farm*, was yet another neighbour. She died in Plumstead in 1921.

Land was cheaper in Southfield Road because it was 'below the railway tracks'. The only development beyond, from the Cape Flats towards Somerset West, was land leased out to coloured farmers who supplied the city and suburbs with vegetables, pigs, and chickens. Initially, this rural part of Plumstead was on the fringe of the *onder-dorp* or lower village of Wynberg, home to poorer working-class and trades people. The wealthier inhabitants lived in the *bo-dorp* or upper village of Wynberg Hill. But this newly opened area was fast becoming fashionable. It attracted professional people who wished to enjoy the pleasures of country life on their smallholdings while they remained within easy reach of the city through road and rail. These affluent property owners, not the least of whom was my grandmother, lost no time in making their demands known to the Wynberg municipality. (4)

Around 1905, Herbert Baker was commissioned to design and build 'Gledsmuir', a three-storey house with a red Marseilles tiled roof, and to landscape the garden. Born in Kent in 1862, Baker had come to South Africa to further his architectural career. His reputation was made in 1900 when he was commissioned by Cecil John Rhodes to renovate and remodel his newly acquired residence at Groote Schuur. As an architect, Baker was already much influenced by the Arts and Crafts Movement in the use of natural materials and traditional building methods. Rhodes then sent him on a study tour of Egypt, Italy and Greece in order that he might add a classical touch to Rhodes' grandiose building projects.

While living at the Cape, Baker designed and built a number of churches and private homes. After Rhodes' death, he moved to the Transvaal where he added to his fame with the construction of some splendid mansions in the fashionable new suburb of Parktown. He also built schools, churches, and public works such as the Union Buildings in Pretoria. By acquiring the services of Baker, the Woods were firmly establishing themselves in Cape society.

The name 'Gledsmuir' was derived from the Gaelic '*Vale of the Hawks or Buzzards*'. *Gled* was a Scots word for a kind of bird of prey, and *muir* meant a heath or moor. There was in fact a village in the East Lothians called Gledsmuir, but there is no knowing if there was any Wood connection to the place.

In addition to an extensive living area, the Woods' house boasted a study, conservatory, and D.J.W.'s pathology laboratory. This took up most of the attic.

31

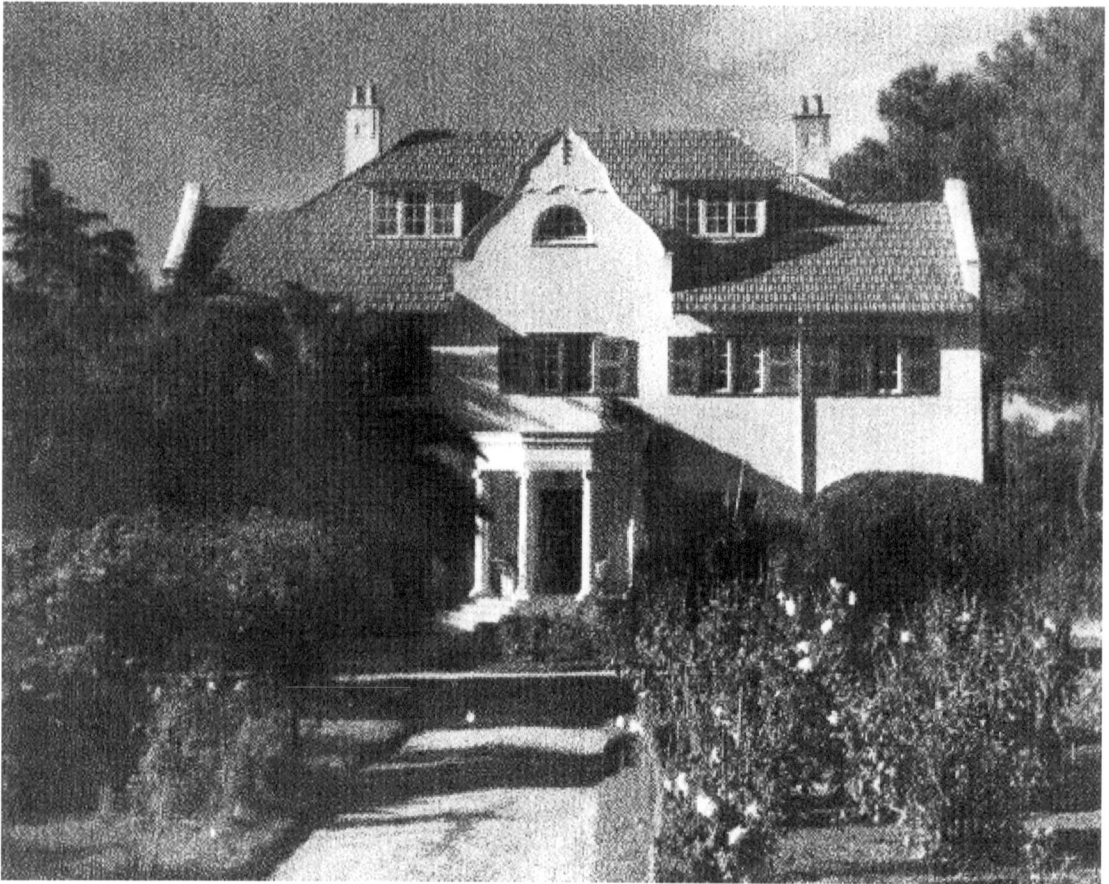

'Gledsmuir', Southfield Road, Plumstead (8)

Outside there was an enormous garden, which included a tennis court, croquet lawn, and a practice golf fairway where Constance used to graze her cows. She much enjoyed the social life and loved to throw parties for which 'Gledsmuir', with its generously proportioned reception rooms, was admirably suited. Their circle of friends included many of the old Cape families such as the Bertrams, Cloetes, and Van der Byls, as well as their neighbours in the professions of law, politics, literature and medicine.

Encompassing about twenty rooms, the house was more than big enough to accommodate the growing family and the much-loved nanny cum governess, Miss Ursula Borlace. Having been recruited by Constance in England, Miss Borlace remained with the Woods until the children were all grown up, holding the fort during Constance's regular trips abroad. When she finally retired, the family set her up to run a small Bed and Breakfast establishment in her native Cornwall.

D.J.W. slept alongside his children, their beds lined up on the east verandah of the house. Wire mesh kept the mosquitoes at bay but only Dad had a light over his bed. Whenever he had a spare moment he would read to them from Kipling, John Buchan,

Dickens, Thacheray, Stalky and Co., Robert Louis Stevenson and the like, making sure that they were well versed in literature from a young age, more especially their Scottish heritage.

All the children were given a good education. Starting off at Star of the Sea in St. James, they went on to Springfield Convent in Wynberg, both Roman Catholic convents. At senior level, Howard attended Rondebosch Boys' High School and then trained as a doctor at Guy's Hospital in London. Harry went to St. Andrew's College, Grahamstown, which by all accounts was pretty rough at the time. The masters gave cuts for any misdemeanour, while fagging and bullying were an accepted part of school life. My father talked about having to clean his prefect's shoes, to iron newspaper to warm his toilet seat each morning, and other unprintable services. Donald spent one year at the Diocesan College (Bishops), Rondebosch, before following Harry to St. Andrew's.

In those days, expatriates still referred to England as 'Home' or 'the Old Country'. English mores ordered their lives whether this was in furnishings and fashion, food and drink, cultural activities and sport, or society magazines and newspapers like *The Illustrated London News* and *The Times*. Howard was the only boy to go overseas because there was no other option for his medical training. For the girls, being 'finished' abroad was an imperative. Madge attended Wynberg Girls' School until 1913. At the age of fourteen, she then accompanied her mother to England and entered Hillcote School for Young Ladies in Eastbourne, Sussex. This institution was run by two ladies 'of gentler birth'. Educated there during the war years, she met her future Australian husband on the voyage home. Patsy went on to study music at the Sorbonne in Paris, while Rosamund stayed with Sir John Evans and his family during her school years in England.

The family spent their summer holidays at 'Little Bourton' in Fish Hoek. This seaside cottage, on the hillside above the road to Simonstown, belonged to Constance and was one of only a handful of houses gracing the bay. The cottage was primitive with no electricity, no running water, and only basic sanitation; but the bunk beds in the back rooms were a great novelty to the young. 'Little Bourton' has remained in the Montgomery family.

At other times Constance would take the children in a dogcart pulled by a stallion called Botha to bathe at Muizenberg. On one memorable occasion, they were returning home via Lakeside when she developed a migraine, which affected her eyesight. She drove the horse too close to the pavement and the wheel hit a lamppost. The cart overturned and the horse galloped off. Donald was dumped in the middle of the road, Rosamund ended up in a hedge, Patsy lost her front teeth, and Constance broke a few ribs. Only Harry remained unscathed.

As the children grew up, friends and neighbours would be invited to play tennis, or croquet on the lawn. Refreshments included iced coffee and sandwiches. Indoors, the dining table was a huge affair and could be swivelled round to form a billiard table, much favoured by the young. Once they married and had children of their own, the extended families would dine regularly on Sundays at 'Gledsmuir'. As a ten year old, Geoff Montgomery remembers feasting on roast sirloin of beef and apple pie, accompanied by large bowls of whipped Jersey cream at every meal. Grandfather had a regular diet of Scottish oat porridge for breakfast.

In addition to his many other interests, D.J.W. was a keen gardener and was inordinately proud of his dahlias and roses. He was also a gifted craftsman. At the weekends, when everyone else was resting after lunch, he would slip away to his workshop behind the house where he did his wood carving, turning and carpentry. He made the most beautiful furniture including the teak cupboards and bookshelves in his consulting rooms, a desk, sideboard, dresser, tables and chairs, and much more. Various members of the male side of the family have inherited these priceless mementoes.

Harry recalled owning a pet monkey, which was always getting into trouble. When it started stealing food from the kitchen, it had to be exchanged for Belgian hares. They were kept in a fowl run where they bred their young underground. One day the floor of D.J.W.'s workshop caved in and he was extremely angry when he fell into a nest of baby hares. When the garage floor also collapsed the hares were banished for good.

Chapter 6
Cars, Trains and Hansom Cabs

D.J.W.'s passport describes him as five foot eight inches in height with blue eyes and brown hair. He started going bald from the age of thirty-five and was left with just a fringe of hair round the back of his head. Quietly spoken and unassuming in demeanour, he still looked forbidding to his grandchildren with his heavy black-rimmed spectacles. In fact, Geoff was overawed by both grandparents who were strictly Victorian in their views and behaviour. None the less, they were adventurous when it came to revolutionary new developments such as the advent of the motor car.

The first motor vehicle arrived in Cape Town in October 1898, although a German Benz had appeared in Johannesburg some months earlier. (1) Alfred Hennessy was the first to take out a driving licence, his car, a Royal Enfield Quad, having the number plate CA1. He was later knighted for his services in founding the Royal Automobile Club and continued to drive his CA1 car until a few days before his death in November 1963. The Royal Enfield was imported by Garlicks Cycle Supply in lower St. George's Street. The story goes that when Hennessy took off from the store, 'he lost control and charged the crowd. An Irish policeman is reputed to have admonished him, saying: "When you intend to go motoring I suggest you leave that machine behind."' (2) Hennessy had to avoid parking in narrow streets as gaping crowds soon gathered around the car. Once he was driving to Green Point when he was held up by a policeman for going over 20 mph. The officer had just arrived from England and was politely informed that as yet there was no speed limit in Cape Town. No charge was laid. (3)

In due course the Divisional Council imposed a speed limit of 8 mph. After much protest the limit was gradually lifted to 30 mph by 1947. The Cape House of Assembly also took note of 'the new menace' and fixed penalties for motoring offences. During the parliamentary debate, John X. Merriman vehemently denounced this innovation. He quoted a verse:

'A buzz, a whizz and a cloud of dust; A ghastly object flashing by; A cold blood-curdling yell, Then silence, and – a smell'. (4)

D.J.W. lost no time in owning one of these 'stinking machines, which scared the locals stiff'. One of the first cars was called the Stanley Steamer. It was an open vehicle, which did in fact let off steam, showering the ladies with wood and coal dust much to their annoyance. Most of the early cars were 'tourers' with a canvas roof, which could be folded down. The sides were open and in bad weather screens of celluloid had to be erected to keep out the wind and rain. (5) By 1912, English visitors had started complaining about the bad driving in Cape Town. One famous motorist, annoyed by the total absence of any attempt to regulate road traffic, was vociferous in denouncing local drivers for being totally ignorant of the rules. (6)

Alfred Hennessy founded the Automobile Club in 1901; and once motoring became popular, races and reliability trials were held to assess the merits of the various models. The first outing, in December 1901, was from Greenmarket Square to Kalk Bay. Over the next few years, day events were held between Cape Town and the Houw Hoek Inn. This was beyond an old wagon halt, Koffiekraal, now called Elgin. (7) When Charlie Rorick, a taxi driver, drove his Gladiator in a reliability trial up Sir Lowry's Pass, the spectators were able to keep up with the car on foot. (8)

Between 1910 and 1914, D.J.W. was the proud owner of three Clement-Talbots. These cars were fast and soon made a name for themselves in competitions, their slogan being 'The Invincible Talbot'. (9) Constance Wood travelled to England to

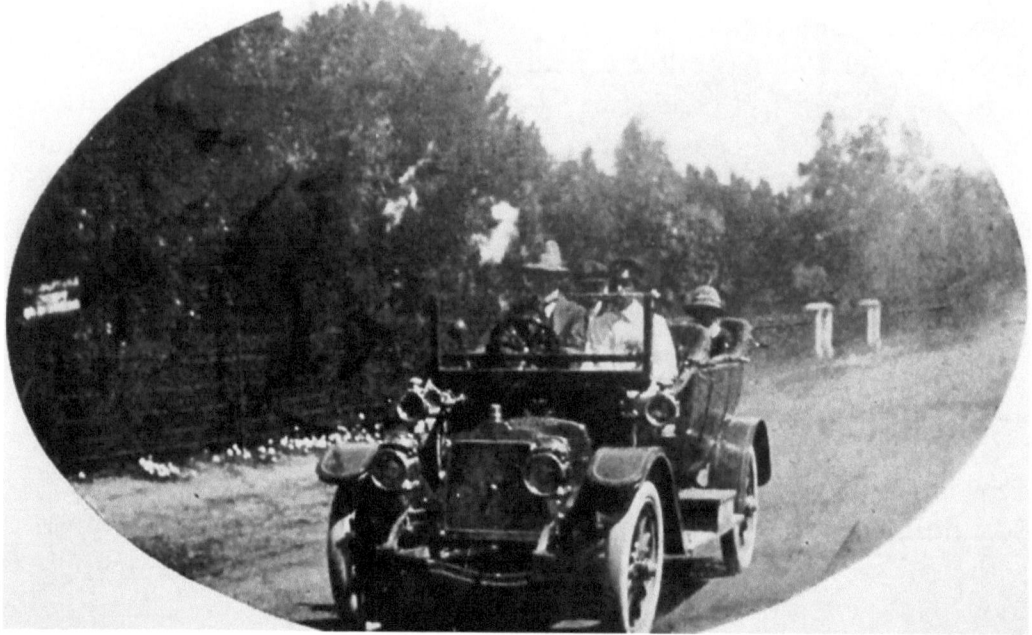

D.J.W. as winner of the Siddeley Cup, 1912, with September (9)

obtain her husband's first Talbot. Togged out in the regulation cap, goggles and motoring coat, he was soon a familiar figure amongst the motoring fraternity. There was one drama when the car's wheel became wedged in the railway line track at the Wetton Road level crossing. The family managed to escape before the car was crushed by a train. The railway paid D.J.W. for the damages.

In October 1912, D.J.W. won the Siddeley Cup in his second Talbot. This was the annual reliability trial from Cape Town to Caledon and back, about one hundred and twenty miles each way. In 1908, J.D. Siddeley, a British manufacturer wishing to promote his Wolseley-Siddeley cars, had offered a floating trophy for a two-day competing event. (10) First held in February 1909, the point-to-point rally took place over timed distances and involved an overnight stop at Caledon. Competitors were each awarded a 1000 mark credit with one mark deducted for every minute out of scheduled time. All seats in the car had to be occupied; and five different engine capacities were selected, ranging from 14 mph to 20 mph in the different classes. (11)

The trial was fairly hazardous as from about two miles out of town there were only dirt roads. Known as 'kalksteen paaie' from the chalky aggregate of the Cape Flats. These roads had been travelled by carts, wagons and carriages over a few hundred years and were littered with every sort of debris including horseshoe nails and bits of steel. The cars carried at least six spare tyres and tubes as punctures were a constant hazard. Even iron studs on the wheels did not help. Each puncture had to be repaired, pumped up and fitted by the driver and his assistant. Jacks were primitive, tyre levers were just two pieces of flat iron, and the tyre pumps were cumbersome and slow in inflating the tubes. At night, the driver had to light his oil-acetylene lamps with matches. Petrol was carried in four-gallon tins, petrol pumps not coming to Cape Town until 1924.

The greatest challenge was to make it up the narrow winding gradients of Sir Lowry's Pass, across the Hottentots Holland range of mountains. The pass had been constructed by the engineer, Charles Mitchell, with the use of convict labour. Opened in July 1830, it was named after Sir Lowry Cole, then Governor of the Cape Colony. (12) Even after the road was widened and tarred in the 1930s, I remember our family car boiling half way up the pass, and having to stop with steam hissing out of the bonnet. We always carried tins of water for such emergencies.

The competitors stayed the night at the Caledon Mineral Baths Hotel and Sanatorium where they were able to enjoy golf, tennis, croquet, bridge, billiards, dancing and hot baths. They returned to Cape Town the next morning after a leisurely breakfast. This was a winner with the ladies. The Caledon Sanatorium had six naturally occurring thermal springs. The rare chalybeate water came gushing out in a continuous flow at 120 degrees Fahrenheit, and had the added healing properties of high ferrous carbonate content. Originally, the Zwartberg springs had been enjoyed by distinguished guests of the DEIC. It was not until the beginning of the 20th century, however, that a three-storey hotel and sanatorium had been built providing luxurious accommodation for three hundred guests.

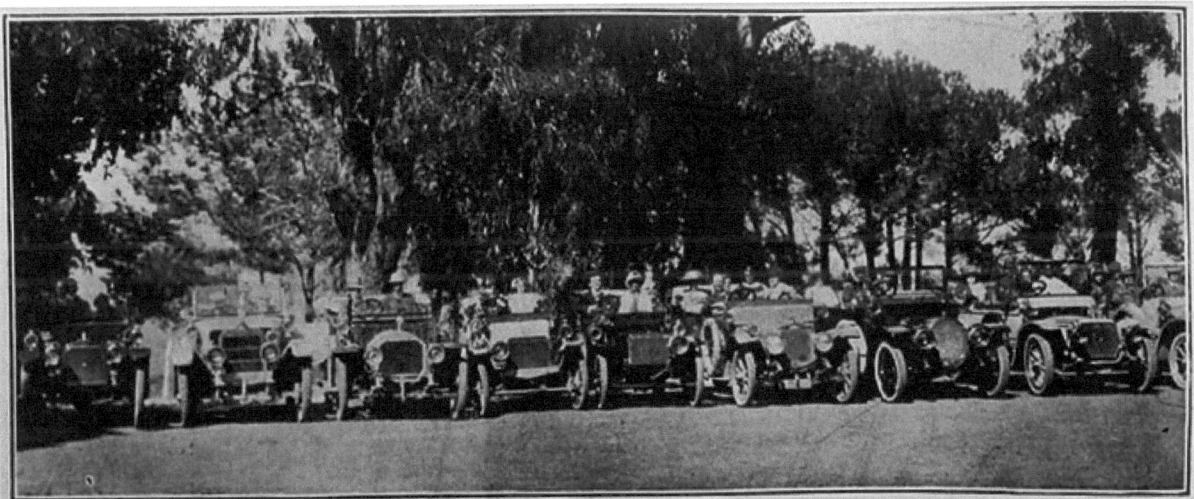

Line up cars for the Siddeley Cup, 1912 (D.J.W. to the extreme left) (10)

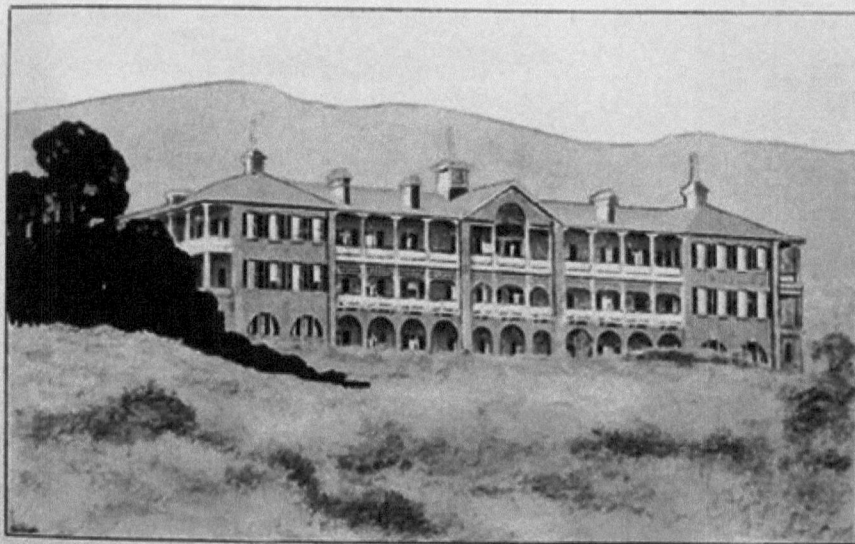

CALEDON BATHS

FOR HEALTH AND PLEASURE.

Natural Radio-Active Thermal Chalybeate Waters.

SANATORIUM HOTEL AND BATHS.

These Waters are World renowned for their Valuable Curative Properties and are highly recommended by the Medical Profession.

The Sanatorium is beautifully situated and is unrivalled for Health and Comfort.

GOLF. TENNIS. CROQUET.

SPLENDID
LARGE SWIMMING BATH
in course of construction.

For the convenience of MOTORISTS:
GARAGE, PETROL STOCKED.

Booklet containing full particulars can be obtained from the Management, the Caledon Baths, Limited, Caledon; or from Messrs. Thos. Cook & Son, Tourist Agents, Cape Town, etc.

Caledon Baths Sanatorium Hotel and Baths (11)

With its fine Victorian furnishings, the spa provided all the comforts of a first class hotel. There was 'good food and perfect service', as well as every facility for health and recreation. These included 'an unusually good library', a large gymnasium, 'a competent masseur', and hospital services with a nurse. Numerous sitting rooms ensured privacy and quiet. There was also a concert hall seating up to six hundred people, with a musicians' gallery and a grand piano. Dances were held here during the summer season. The railway line to Caledon had been opened in 1902 and the trip from Cape Town had previously taken about two hours by rail, or five by cart; but by 1912 the road was said to be good. (13)

D.J.W.'s second Talbot had a 12 horsepower engine, and was capable of reaching 60 mph. Family tradition claims that in winning the Siddeley Cup race in 1912, it covered the distance to Caledon at an average of twenty-five miles to the gallon. The cup was three feet high and was presented together with a gold plaque. Alfred Hennessy came third in his 20hp Standard. No race was held in 1913 and the last competition took place in 1914. The winner was A. B. Godbold, another Wood family friend, driving a 9.5 hp Standard. This time D.J.W. came fifth in his 12hp Talbot. (14) The Siddeley Cup trials were not held during the Great War due to fuel restrictions. The last one in November 1914 and was won by the winner of the 1909 event, C.F. Spilhaus in his Wolseley.

After the war, Siddeley amalgamated with Armstrong-Whitworth to build the Armstrong Siddeley car. They also made aeroplanes. In 1935, Siddeley's interests were bought by Tommy (Sir Thomas) Sopwith, who went on to create the famous Hawker Hurricane fighter planes of World War II. (15)

In 1913, a four cylinder 25hp Talbot, highly tuned, lightened, and fitted with a racing body, was driven by Percy Lambert to become the first car to cover 100 miles an hour at Brooklands Race Track. (16) The following year Constance Wood went to England to buy the new model, their third Talbot. She was accompanied by their coloured chauffeur, September. The car cost about seven hundred and fifty pounds, a lot of money in those days. Streamlined, it weighed about two tons, had a folding hood, a long smooth touring body, and an array of brass fittings. Constance was fed up because when September tried it out at Brooklands it only reached between 75 and 85 mph instead of the expected 100. The manufacturers agreed to reduce the price even though the car was weighed down with all its extra accoutrements.

Poor September had to learn to drive the Talbot in London. He was extremely nervous and stopped once to let the traffic pass by. Immediately, a policeman marched up and asked his name. "Cornelius Aurelius Peter September" was the reply. "None of your lip, darkie", snarled the bobby, "You can't drive like that here. Move on." The car caused a sensation in Cape Town, attracting crowds of admirers, and was with the family for sixteen years. Later on it was used by a funeral company as a hearse.

September was a large fat man who loved to play the violin. He played extremely badly; but my father, Harry, enjoyed sitting and listening to him during his lunch break and sharing in a good conversation. With the outbreak of World War I, September was taken on as a driver in a Guards Regiment in England. He was very sad about leaving the Wood family, though, saying how much he would miss seeing Miss Patsy's beautiful golden curls. Harry was so upset that he knocked Patsy down and cut off some of her ringlets as a parting present. He got into terrible trouble as a result. Great was the excitement when September returned from the war with his smart uniform and army equipment.

On one occasion, as D.J.W. came rollicking down Sir Lowry's Pass in one of his Talbots, he was held up by Alfred Hennessy blocking the narrow road. September was having none of this. When they got close he took out a revolver and fired it in the air, making an awful racket. Much alarmed that a tyre had blown, Hennessy drew over to the side of the road to inspect the damage, allowing D.J.W. to go sailing past. September was also required to ferry the young to and fro from dances, until such time as they obtained their own driving licenses. The boys all sported motorbikes and although the roads were not all that good there was not much traffic. Harry

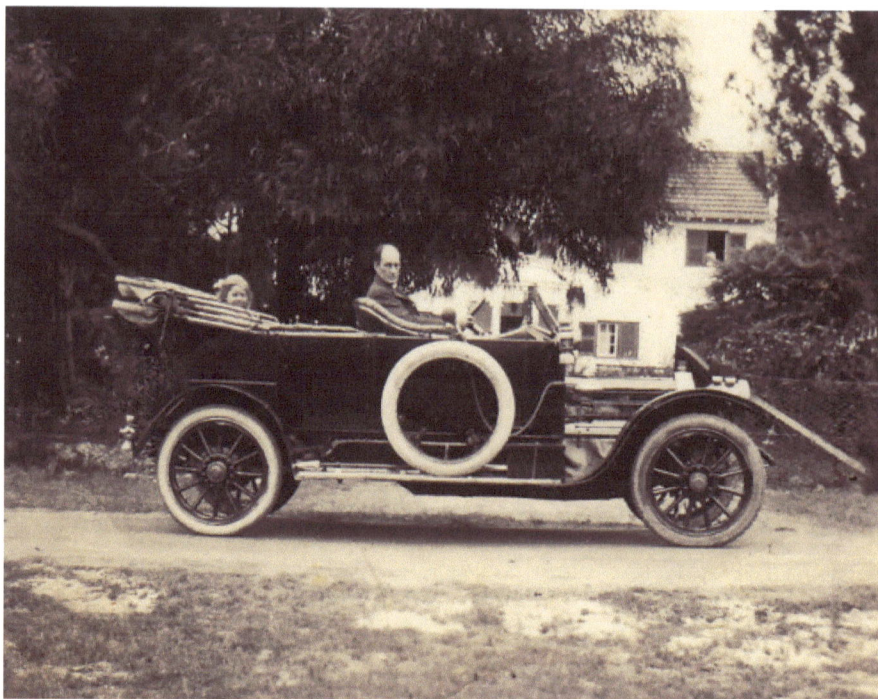

D.J.Wood with one of his cars and a young daughter (12)

regularly raced to Fish Hoek on his Harley Davidson, claiming to be able to make the trip from Retreat in ten minutes.

Over the years, D.J.W. owned a good number of other cars from a 1910 Sunbeam, Essex, Hudson and a bull-nosed Morris, painted canary yellow, to a Studebaker straight eight tourer. All the vehicles were open while the Morris had a dickey seat at the back, much favoured by grandchildren. The Studebaker was a 1932 model with a top speed of 60 mph.

When operating D.J.W. always used public transport for fear that the stress and strain of driving his car would interfere with the delicate touch required for intra-ocular surgery. (17) The suburban railway line had been completed as far Wynberg in April 1864, after much controversy, petitioning, financial crises and bureaucratic hold-ups. Wynberg village then became a dormitory suburb of Cape Town. When the line was extended to the False Bay coast and Simonstown in 1884, a stopping place was made two km. beyond Wynberg to handle the fruit, grapes and other agricultural produce from surrounding farms and the Constantia Valley. A wood and iron building was erected and the station was named Plumstead after the village. (18) At the turn of the century, the advent of residences 'below the line' led to Plumstead station becoming popular with professional men commuting to Cape Town, now able to travel quickly and easily into work.

On arriving at Cape Town station, D.J.W. would take a hansom cab or taxi to the New Somerset Hospital in Green Point, or the Hof Street Nursing Home in Oranjezicht. This was a former farm on the lower slopes of Table Mountain. At Hof Street he was in partnership with other surgeons and it was there that he operated on his private patients. As his granddaughter, I was treated royally when I had my appendix removed at Hof Street Nursing Home as late as 1950.

The horse-drawn hansom cabs had long plied their trade in the city, two hundred being licensed by 1891. (19) They charged half-a-crown for the first hour and a florin thereafter. The Malay stand was at the bottom of Adderley Street near the railway station, while Irish cab drivers catered for a select clientele of Parliamentarians. The most lucrative stand was outside the Mount Nelson Hotel. Lawrence G. Green describes red-fezzed Malay drivers urging their horses to reach a top speed of seven miles an hour, their huge wooden wheels trundling over the Dock Road cobblestones. Some horses sported straw hats to protect them from the sun, their ears protruding through holes. The cabs all had names, too, like 'Alabama', 'Happy Go Lucky' and 'Spes Bona'. (20)

The cab trade reached its peak servicing the troop trains during the Anglo-Boer War. Thereafter they could not compete with the trams or the motorised taxis that followed. (21) By 1911 there were about five hundred taxis in Cape Town, the speed limit having been raised to ten miles an hour. In vain did the cab drivers hold protest meetings, thinking that taxis would soon go out of fashion. In Cape Town the pedestrians had always been a nuisance as they assumed right of way on the roads. When the cab drivers finally became reconciled to cars, they struggled even more to negotiate the over-crowded streets. (22)

Chapter 7
Bottled Eyes and Brains

The top floor or attic at 'Gledsmuir' was largely taken up by D.J.W.'s pathology laboratory with a couple of small bedrooms for Madge, Howard and Nanny. Piles of dusty old books that had come from Scotland were stacked along the passage, many in French. The lab itself had windows in the roof along one side, while the opposite wall was lined with row upon row of shelves stacked with a mass of small bottles and glass dishes holding bits and pieces of eyes. All were carefully labelled, some awaiting examination. The pathology specimens were preserved in formalin, providing a pervasive smell to which D.J.W. alone seemed impervious. It was not unknown for a bottled eye to be displayed on the dining room table while the family ate their meal. They would be treated to a full account of its origin and as to why it was of particular interest.

D.J.W.'s usual practice was to retire to his lab after dinner each evening. If any of the young joined him while he was working, they would be invited to admire a newly preserved eye accompanied by a typical comment: "Yes, old Mrs. So and So's. Written to London to match it. I hope the replacement will be here soon." A large Zeiss microscope was more to the boys' liking. They kept themselves amused by using it to study pond life. This they collected in glass jars from the vlei at the bottom of Southfield Road. They used tin baths carried on their heads as boats. Otherwise they made canoes of corrugated iron nailed to two long planks of wood. These invariably sank but the vlei was shallow at the edges.

According to Geoff Montgomery, his grandfather invented his own surgical knife. This was mounted on a base with various controls that could be manipulated to produce a section the equivalent of one cell in thickness for examination. The newly discovered collection of his photographic glass plates at Groote Schuur Hospital seem to bear this out. D.J.W. personally sectioned and stained every piece of tissue that he removed from patients to add to his collection of pathology specimens. The slides were all carefully mounted and meticulously annotated with his diagnosis, as well as references to any procedures, which had been carried out. After his death, the fact that he had devoted all his spare time to increasing his knowledge of the eye, its physiology, anatomy and disorders, was universally acclaimed. His collection of ocular specimens was bequethed to the Department of Ophthalmology at Groote Schuur and was regarded as textbook material for students for many years afterwards.

Long wooden trays, with eight sealed glass dishes containing pathology specimens, each sunk separately into round cavities, are now in the Medical Museum at Green Point, Cape Town, and in the Ophthalmology Museum in the Out Patient Department at Groote Schuur. The trays were made by D.J.W. himself. Examples of his handwritten notes on the lids of the dishes, some rather worn, have been deciphered as:

- 19 III 1905. Rt. Eye. Mrs Meredith. Visual failure 1 month. V. 6/9. Large sharp edged detachment of lower part of fundus. Recurrence of growth. Spindle celled Sarcoma partly fragmented.

- Glaucoma. Perforating ulcer resulting in sudden fall of tension and three large haemorrhages. Mrs. Collins 1918.

- J4 Wound by stick. Cornea adherent to remains of Lens. Recurrent abrasion. Excised for pain. Mrs Brown. 1920.

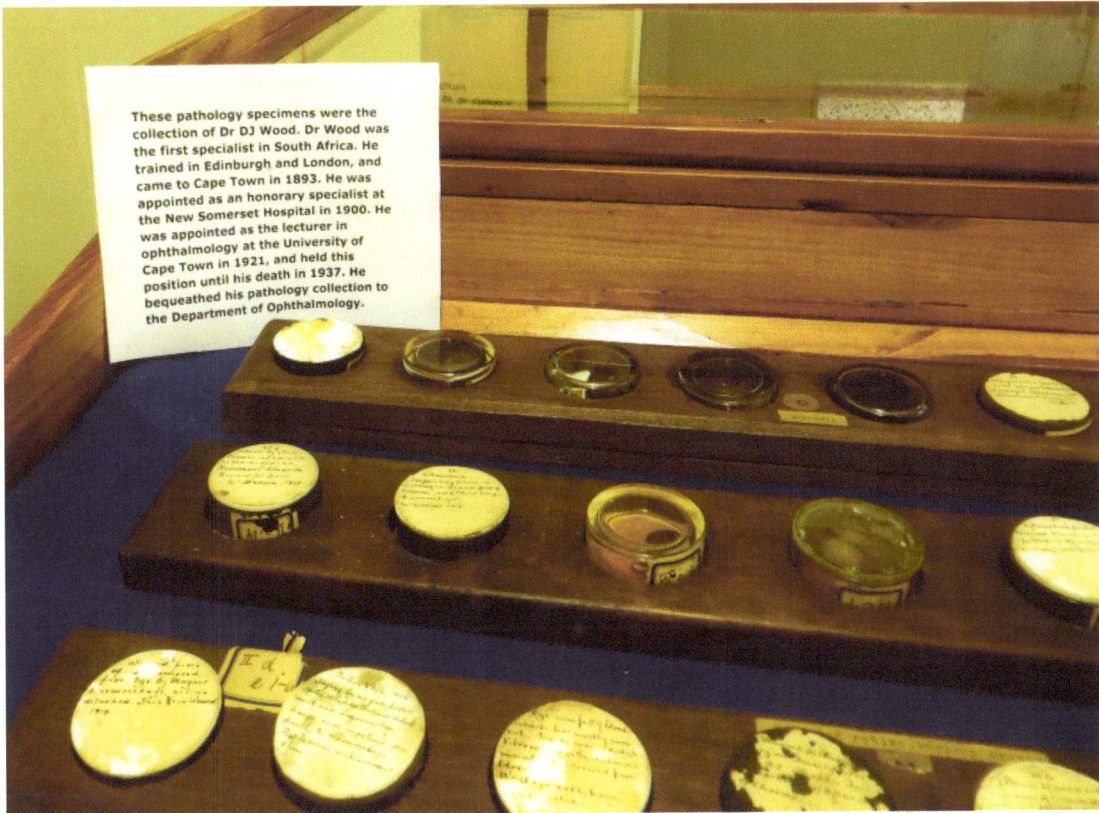

These pathology specimens were the collection of Dr DJ Wood. Dr Wood was the first specialist in South Africa. He trained in Edinburgh and London, and came to Cape Town in 1893. He was appointed as an honorary specialist at the New Somerset Hospital in 1900. He was appointed as the lecturer in ophthalmology at the University of Cape Town in 1921, and held this position until his death in 1937. He bequeathed his pathology collection to the Department of Ophthalmology.

D.J.W.'s trays of pathogenic specimens (13)

- Eye from which a large fragment was removed three weeks previously. Wound in sclera. Six days in Eye. Taylor. 1921.

- Joan Vlok. Injury by airgun pellet. Optic atrophy, retinal detachment and degeneration. Large scar due partly to haemorrhage. Post-mortem displacement of lens.

- J.E. Turner Dr. Dreyer's patient. Sept. 1935. Pigmented Sarcoma. Complaint - loss of outer field of vision.

- Q3 Bulging of Pseudo cornea Ophth. neon. Cupping of O.D.

Part of the laboratory was given over to photography and included a sink. Shutters against the windows could be closed to create a dark room. In his D.J. Wood Memorial Lecture in 1977, Professor Justin L. van Selm said that over forty years later, Wood's micro-photography of sections of the human eye was still considered to be quite outstanding. This was particularly so when one realized that he photographed, developed and printed the pictures using the unsophisticated equipment available at the time. (1)

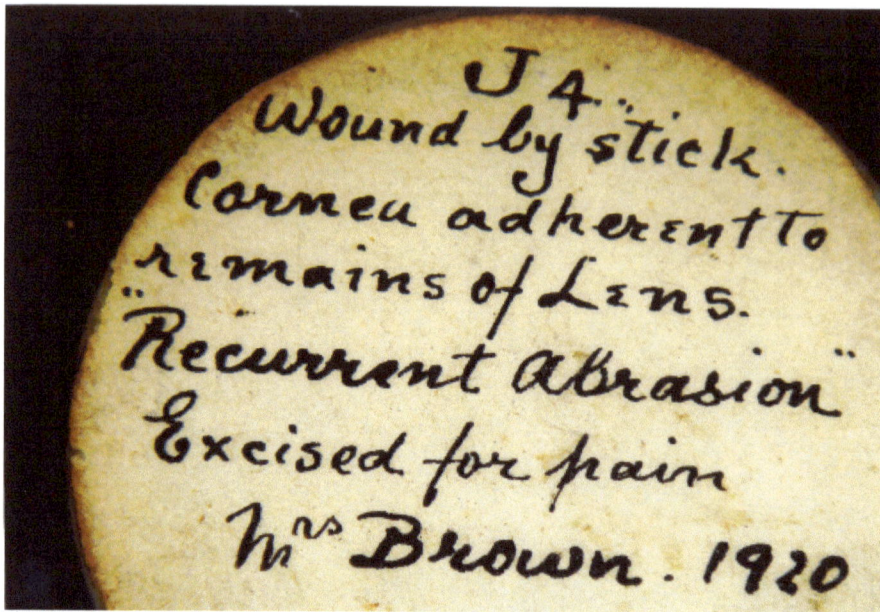

Label on pathogenic specimen of Mrs. Brown, 1920. (14)

A micro-photograph is a photograph taken through a microscope or similar device to show a magnified image of an item such as a prepared section of an eye mounted on a slide. The camera would have been attached to the miscroscope. The glass photographic plate could be projected using a magic lantern or else printed as a photograph. (2) John B. Dancer (1812-1887), a Manchester optician and instrument maker, was one of the pioneers in this field and D.J.W. would have been familiar with his work. Photographic dry glass plates, which had replaced the earlier wet glass plates, preceded film as a photographic medium. The dry plates, coated with a light-sensitive emulsion of silver salts, were commonly used between the 1880s and the 1920s, although D.J.W. continued using them to the end of his life. Not only did they produce high quality images, ideal in research, but they were extremely stable, as is evident from his collection, now about eighty years old.

In this electronic and digital era it is amazing to see the fine detail of cells, blood vessels, tissues, nerve fibres, and membranes which D.J.W. managed to achieve in minute sections of diseased and damaged eyes. His micro-photographs were accompanied by precise information regarding the pathological examination of the specimen. This included the process by which the sections had been sliced, the way they had been treated with preservatives and stained, and the levels of magnification. From the 1920s on, D.J.W.'s papers on a wide variety of clinical cases appeared almost annually in the *British Journal of Ophthalmology (BJO)*, and the majority were liberally illustrated with examples of his photographic genius. As the years progressed the illustrations became ever more sophisticated, being greatly enhanced by modern printing technology not then available in South Africa. (3)

With his enquiring mind and broad medical training, D.J.W's research interests extended far beyond eyes. On one occasion a notorious murderer was hanged in Roeland Street jail. Grandfather persuaded the Governor to give him the man's brain, which he wanted to study to see if he could detect any abnormalities. One Friday afternoon a brown paper bag with the brain was delivered to his rooms, but he forgot to take it home. Come Monday he took his precious parcel to the train, placed it in the luggage rack and settled down to read his newspaper. By the time the rush hour train had reached Mowbray he was surprised to see that his fellow passengers had abandoned the carriage. When he arrived home he was told by his wife to get that stinking thing out of the house or else she would leave forthwith. It was only then that he noticed the smell. The brain was hastily buried, although Donald remembered another human brain being preserved in formalin in a pyrex dish with a lid on it.

D.J.W.'s absent-mindedness caused other problems too. On numerous occasions the telephone at 'Gledsmuir' would ring around 5.30 p.m. The doctor was waiting at Plumstead station and wanted someone to come and fetch him. He would then be reminded that he had taken his car to work but had forgotten that he had left it parked in Church Square.

Church Square had an interesting history in that the Slave Lodge, built by the Dutch burghers in the late 17th century, was originally located diagonally opposite to D.J.W.'s consulting rooms in the National Mutual Buildings. At that time the square served as a slave market, and slaves remained living in the Lodge until 1811. Thereafter, the government used the building as the Cape Supreme Court, the library and the post office.

Directly opposite D.J.W.'s rooms was the 'Groote Kerk', the mother church of the Dutch Reformed Church (Nederduitse Gereformeerde Kerk), the established church of the Colony. Consecrated in 1704, it is the oldest existing church in southern Africa. The square was not officially called 'Kerkplijn' or Church Square until the late 18th century. When D.J.W. first went there, the 'slave tree' still existed on the corner with Spin Street. Originally, it was the place under which the slaves were auctioned. Later, they would sit beside their masters' carriages in the shade of the old fir tree waiting for the church service to end. (4) The tree was removed in 1916 and the square was reduced in size over the years to accommodate a cemetery. It later became a convenient parking place for the new-fangled motor cars.

Chapter 8
Tinus de Jongh, Medical Artist

Another of D.J.W.'s achievements was in obtaining the services of a struggling young artist, Tinus De Jongh (Jong), to paint pictures of fundus pathology and the inner eye for teaching purposes at the new University of Cape Town Medical School (UCT). The fundus is the observed interior surface of the eye. Some of these remarkable illustrations were still being used in the ophthalmology department many years later.

Before long Tinus de Jongh became popular as a landscape painter of Western Cape scenery. However, his earlier work as the first medical artist in South Africa has received scant recognition. This was probably because most of his medical watercolours were locked away in a storeroom at Groote Schuur Hospital for many years and have never been seen by the public. Now framed, the paintings might be thought to be of limited interest; but with their vibrant ochre colouring and detailed anatomical depictions of eyes, they seem to simulate modern art, and are of immense historical value.

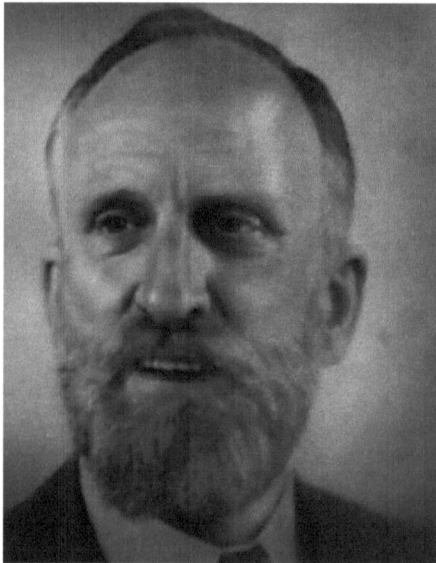

Tinus de Jongh (15)

Born in Amsterdam in the Netherlands in 1885, Marthinus 'Tinus' Johannes De Jongh showed his artistic talent when young. At the age of eleven he was given permission by the Rijks Museum to copy works of 'the Golden Age of Dutch Art' of the 17th century. Yet his parents forbade him to make a formal study of art and so he began work with a firm of decorators. This lasted two years before he embarked on painting as a full-time career. Largely self-taught, he started with street scenes, interiors and landscapes in the formal style of the Amsterdam tradition. At fifteen he painted his first major work in oils depicting a blacksmith's workshop. As he gained local recognition, buyers of his paintings included the Stedelike Museum.

In 1921, De Jongh emigrated to South Africa. His wife and three young children followed six months later. They began life at the Cape in a one-roomed cottage in Diep River, but later settled in Rondebosch. In the beginning De Jongh continued with his muted Dutch style of painting, focusing on local street scenes and views; but the vibrancy of colours, bright light and magnificent scenery of his new surroundings was soon reflected in his art. At weekends his love of nature drove

46

him to hike throughout the Cape Peninsula, inspiring him to embark on his distinctive landscapes. He was accompanied by his only son, Gabriel. When Tinus acquired a car, his travels took him further afield in the Western Cape and beyond. This led to a wealth of paintings of mountain scenery, with jagged peaks bathed in pastel colours by the setting sun, and verdant tree-lined valleys with their winding rivers and gabled, white-washed farmhouses. Gabriel also became a noted South African artist, following his father in much the same style of painting. (1)

De Jongh's colourful Cape landscapes were soon in popular demand while his paintings of city scenes were bought by banks, private institutions and patrons of the arts. His first public commission, to paint the Houses of Parliament, was hung in the office of the High Commissioner of South Africa in London. His etchings sold in hundreds and were the subject of the first case of art forgery in South Africa. Louis Woolf, a Cape Town art dealer, handled the sale of the etchings. After De Jongh moved to Bloemfontein, Woolf forged the artist's signature on thousands more of these works. When taken to court, Woolf argued that De Jongh had granted him permission; but he was found guilty in what became a scandalous affair covering inches in the daily newspapers. (2)

Esme Berman believes that the popularity of Tinus De Jongh's paintings with the wider buying public was due to their being 'sumptuous in scale, local in content, descriptive in character, traditional in style and bright in colour'. She also notes that he was an inveterate pipe-smoker, and that 'his friends joked that his pipe was even more essential to his working habits than his brush'. (3) His paintings became collector's items after his death from lung cancer in Bloemfontein, in 1942.

In 1923, while De Jongh was still struggling to make a living as an artist at the Cape, he was commissioned by the faculty Heads of the Departments of Gynaecology and Ophthalmology at UCT to paint a series of medical illustrations for teaching purposes. Medical illustrations have a long history in the art world, reaching far back into antiquity, although early works tended to be imaginative with minimal if any medical knowledge. (4) The modern understanding of medical art was not realized until the Renaissance in Italy led by Leonardo da Vinci (1452-1519). Not only did he have formal training in anatomy, but he was given permission to dissect human corpses so that his scientific drawings were based on a precise examination of body parts. Michelangelo (1475-1564) also carried out dissections over many years in order to improve his understanding of human anatomy, as exemplified in his paintings and sculptures. (5) Applied medical art was only formalised as a profession, in America, in the early 20th century. (6)

At the start of his brief career as a medical artist in the Ophthalmology Department, De Jongh copied pictures from textbooks or the work of others,

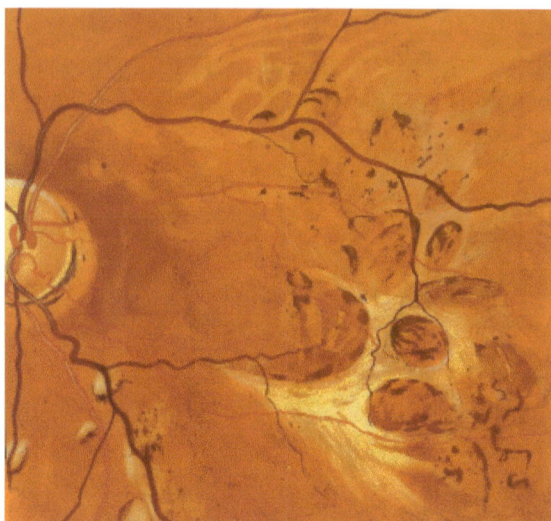
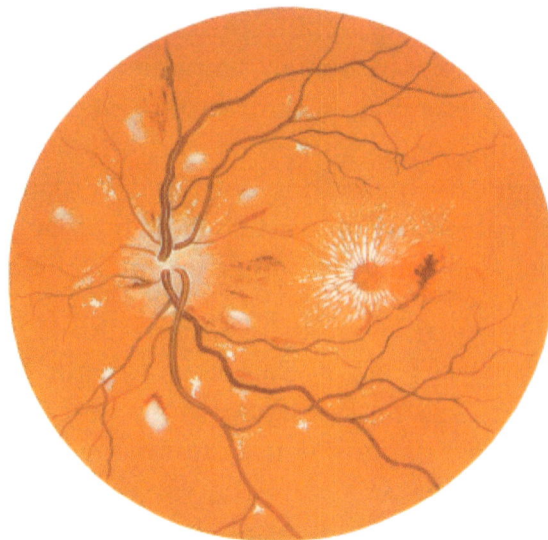

Unsigned painting by Tinus de Jongh
'Retinitis Proliferans' (16)

Unsigned painting by Tinus de Jongh of
'Albumenuric Retinitis Pregnancy' (17)

including my grandfather. Once D.J.W. had taught him how to use an ophthalmoscope, the instrument used to see the back of the eye, his watercolour paintings of diseases of the fundus were original, and the only ones he deigned to sign. His concern to record every detail with the clarity and precision of a camera is reflected in his work in the medical field.

Three of De Jongh's largest fundus paintings, in ochre colouring and with a bold signature, hang in the passage of the Department of Ophthalmology in the original building of the Groote Schuur Hospital. One is untitled but the other two are called 'Choroidal Tubercle' and 'Thrombosis of Retinal Vein'. Professor Colin Cook, Head of the Department, has had the collection of 21 unsigned De Jongh paintings framed, together with another signed one, and they hang in the seminar room, library and passage of the D4 wing of the hospital. The Gynaecology Department also has a small collection of black and white medical illustrations hanging in their passage, signed by De Jongh.

Four large paintings by D.J.W. comprise part of the Ophthalmology collection and have been hung in the passage. Only one is signed but the style, the artistic technique, and the texture of paper are different from those of De Jongh's watercolours and are undoubtedly D.J.W.'s work. In the library there is a small finely detailed painting initialled by him, too, entitled 'Raised sub-retinal exudate. H.P. Left eye'. Two even smaller paintings are unsigned but are in the same style and have been hung together. They are given as Sister Magdalene, January – May 1930.

In May 2013, Professor Tony Murray, former Head of the Department, unearthed another box of ten watercolour paintings in the storeroom, some signed D.J.W., but all done by him. They are rather faded but as works of art, and with the attention to detail, they are amazing. Treasure indeed. These have now been reframed and are hanging in the D4 library. A number were published with his papers in the *BJO*. (See Appendix 6 for a list of the paintings.)

D.J.W. also made many demonstration drawings and models of the inner eye. These were carefully annotated for teaching purposes when he became the first lecturer in Ophthalmology at UCT. (7) This was painstaking work so that it must have been a relief to hand some of it over to De Jongh.

✧

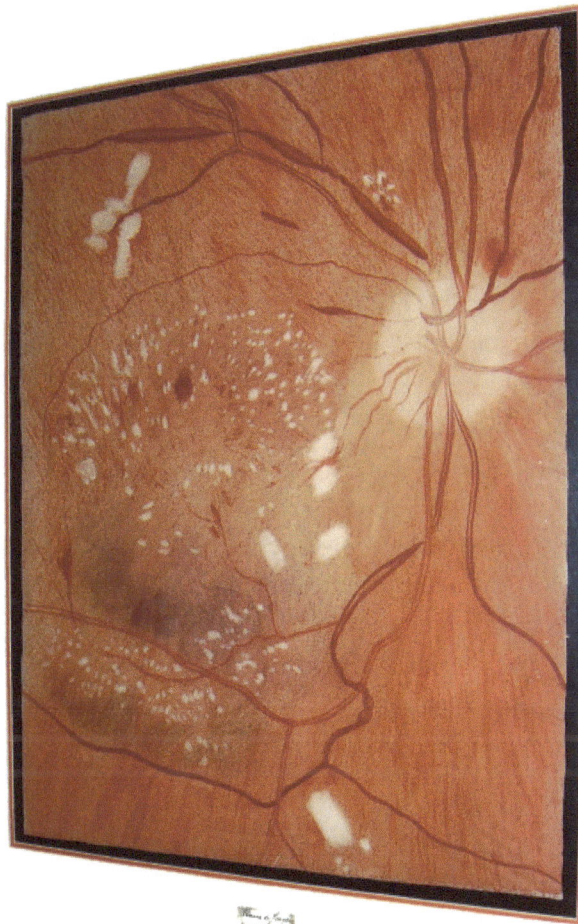

Signed fundus painting by Tinus de Jongh (18)

PART 3: CONSTANCE CLARA WOOD

Chapter 9
Family and Farming

Constance Clara Cooke was born on 27th November 1870 in the Cotwolds hamlet of Cropredy, England. This was situated just north of Banbury in Oxfordshire. Nearby is the larger village of Great Bourton, which is sometimes given as her birthplace. Although anything but sentimental by nature, she named her seaside cottage at Fish Hoek, 'Little Bourton', retaining a tenuous link with her roots at 'Home'. Her father, John Cooke, was the village squire. He was born about 1822 in Warwick, Warwickshire. According to the 1861 census he owned 220 acres of land. Constance's mother, Sarah Muckley, came from Great Bourton but nothing more is known about her except that she was born around 1831.

The Cooke family must have been quite well off as they employed six men and two boys on the farm, as well as a house servant and dairymaid. Then in 1871, Constance's father had a fatal riding accident when trying to jump a high stone wall while out hunting. He was reputed to be a 'two bottle a day' man but what was in the bottle was never said. (1)

Constance was the youngest of five siblings. Mary, the eldest, was born about 1855. She was followed by Edith (born c.1857), Arthur (born c.1859), Charles (born c.1867) and Constance. She was not yet a year old when her father died. The family were left in straightened circumstances and so she was adopted by Charles Duffel Faulkner (born 1827) and his wife Elizabeth. He was the local coroner and solicitor, and they had no children of their own. The 1881 census has Sarah Cooke, a widow, as head of her household. She was living with her daughter, Mary, who was employed locally as a governess. Charles was also still at home; but Constance, who had initially received private tuition with the Faulkners, had been sent to boarding school in Leamington.

Ten years later, the next census has Constance staying with her married sister, Edith, in Portsmouth. Duffel Faulkner had died in the interim. Nothing more is known about her background except that in her early twenties she was diagnosed as having a delicate chest. Family tradition regards this as nonsense as she never developed any further symptoms and lived an extremely energetic and full life. At the time, however, being sent to a drier climate was standard practice for those thought to be in danger of contracting tuberculosis. Like her father she was high-spirited, and shipping her off to South Africa as a teacher might well have been a fashionable way of relieving her family of a difficult charge, or, at the least, an uncertain future. At any rate her shipboard romance with D.J.W. solved any future problems. Howard, her eldest son, was given the name Faulkner in appreciation of all her adoptive father had done for her.

After moving to South Africa, the only known contact Constance had with her family was in 1922 when she took Donald, her youngest son, on one of her many trips to England. He turned ten while on board and had vivid memories of the voyage. This included swimming in a canvas bath on the foredeck and of driving around Tenerife in an old taxi. One of the purposes of this particular visit was to bring back spare parts for an enormous Eagle Range coal stove that dominated the kitchen. It had two ovens, one for roasting and one for baking, and it had to be lit at 4 a.m. every day.

During this visit Donald met Uncle Charlie, his mother's brother, who was 'a bit of a tippler' and the black sheep of the family. Uncle Charlie was a

Constance Clara Wood at 'Gledsmuir' (19)

gifted craftsman who made magnificent models of ships and the like. He presented Donald with a much treasured foot long model of a British field gun replete with horses in harness. Constance took rooms in the Prince of Wales Mansions opposite Battersea Park, and here Donald enjoyed endless games of cricket with his cousins. Once, after he had made a spectacular catch, his uncle presented him with a leather cricket ball and bat. Much to Donald's delight, the bat was signed by the famous cricketer, J.B. Hobbs, whose sporting goods shop was just down the road. 'Jack' Hobbs played for England in sixty-one Test matches between 1908 and 1930, and is still regarded as one of the best batsmen of all time. He was the first professional cricketer to be knighted, in 1953.

Following her marriage in 1895, Constance became a formidable figure in her own right, making a significant contribution both in her local community and in the wider society. In 1913 she was listed among the prominent women in South Africa. (2) Independent, capable and forever active, she took full charge of running the home and extensive property. An excellent cook herself, she had a large staff including a Norwegian cook, a scullery girl, and a maid with her own parlour, not to mention

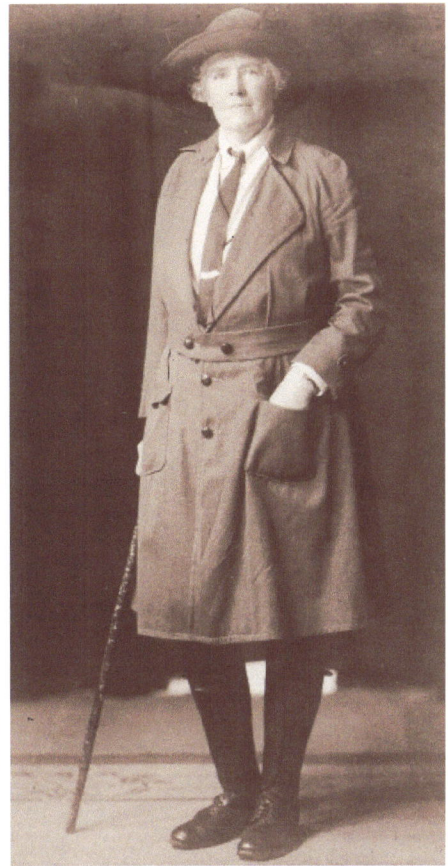

the chauffeur and a team of gardeners and farm labourers. The Norwegian cook later went on to work in Government House and was replaced by African male cooks. But Constance needed to be perpetually occupied and so she launched into poultry farming. She soon had hundreds of chickens, as well as geese, turkeys and ducks, with two duck ponds. One year she won first prize at the Rosebank Show with a large white turkey that had turned up out of the blue.

In 1916, her animal husbandry became more serious when she established her own Jersey cattle herd, importing pedigreed stock direct from Jersey in the Channel Islands. For many years the dairy was run under the name of Jersey Creamery. Dressed in riding breeches and gaiters, she rose early every morning to supervise the milking of her cows. This was long before the days of milking machines and it was all done by hand. In my father's dairy I still remember the sound of milk squirting into buckets, and the scraping of the three-pronged metal stools on the cement floor as the milkmen moved from cow to cow, not forgetting the rich smell of cow dung. In the late afternoon granny would still be found churning butter from the rich Jersey cream. She used one of those old wooden churns, turning a handle, which operated paddles inside. After this the buttermilk had to be drained off and the butter scraped out.

Constance supplied the Lewis Simms store around the corner from Longmarket Street, Cape Town. (3) They specialised in poultry and fish and she delivered the fresh produce herself. She had a dogcart and trap pulled by a Basuto pony, which nipped along at a merry pace. Shortly after Howard had graduated as a doctor from Guy's Hospital in London, he accompanied her on one of her deliveries. Very dignified, he was given a basket of four ducks to take to the shop. The bottom fell out of the basket and the ducks scattered down the street in every direction. They were finally rounded up but poor Howard was much mortified. His mother also supplied Jersey cream to Lewis Simms by train. A staff member once phoned to say that they had found a mouse floating in one of her cream cans. He received short shrift. "What's the matter," she said, "Why can't you take it out?"

In the early years of motoring at the Cape there were few women drivers. Unfazed, Constance exchanged her dogcart and pony for a Ford motor car. One day, as she was busy working in the garden, a policeman arrived with a summons for her to appear in court. She had failed to get her new car licensed. The magistrate happened to be a friend of hers and so the hapless policeman was instructed to "Tell Mr. Elliott at the registration office to mind his own business, and if you don't go I will squirt you with water". And he left hastily. In later years, she gave up driving herself. With a now elderly September at the wheel, she was an extremely nervous passenger and became hysterical if he went over 25mph. If he dared exceed 30 mph she would shout "Slow down, slow down!"

Constance suffered from high blood pressure and was subject to outbursts of temper. In those days the only treatment was to bleed the patient to try and relieve the pressure. Geoff remembers basins of blood being carried out of her bedroom. Forthright in manner and with a sharp tongue, she is said to have bullied her husband unmercifully. Nor did she suffer fools gladly, never hesitating to speak her mind so that people walked warily in her presence.

Undoubtedly, she was endowed with extraordinary reserves of intellectual and physical stamina. But the physical toughness of her complex persona was combined with a degree of sensual magnetism, which could be mistaken for unladylike immodesty not commensurate with the prevailing mores of the time. Although she had little patience with most other women, she associated freely with men and over the years gave financial support to a number of elderly gentlemen friends who had fallen on hard times. She was impervious to gossip in certain prudish sections of the community.

Despite any shortcomings, Constance had a strong sense of justice for the needy, and was involved in numerous good works. She was a committee member of the Seamen's Institute, but her major project was organising soup kitchens across the Cape Flats, mostly at her own expense. Plumstead was situated on the western edge of this huge, windswept area of sand dunes and marshland between the Cape

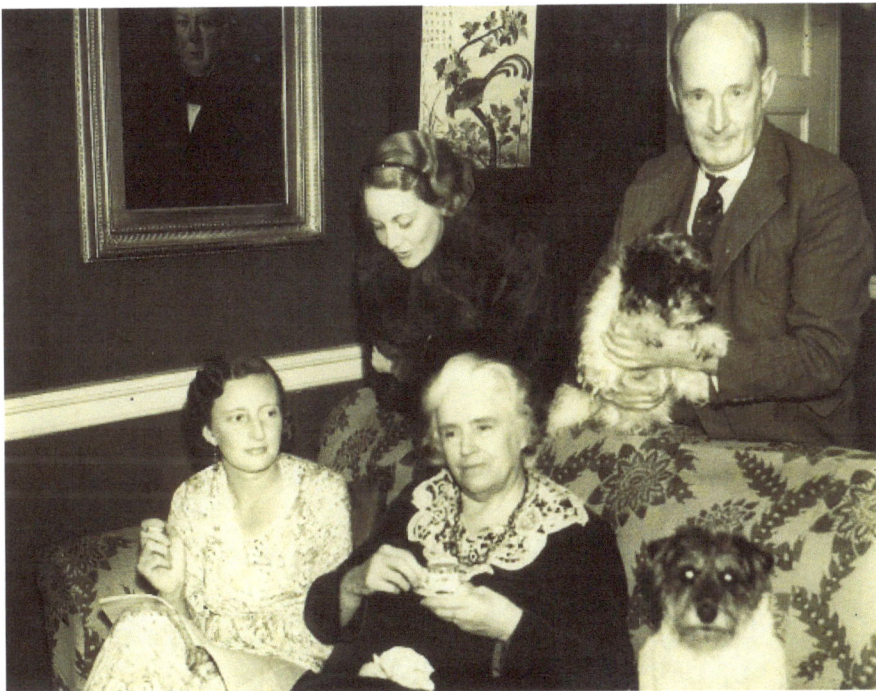

Dr. D.J. Wood and Constance Wood with Patsy and Rosamund (20)

53

Peninsula and the Hottentots Holland mountains. Early Dutch settlers called it the 'Kaapsche Duine' or 'Zand Vlakte'. Their wagons had been forced to avoid the treacherous soft sand by travelling via the 'Hardekraaltjie uitspan', present-day Bellville, where the ground was firmer. By the middle of the 19th century small farmers, including a band of German settlers, had begun to graze cattle and to grow vegetables in the area to feed the Capetonians. In the 1880s, the Forestry Department tried to bind the sand by planting the fast-growing Australian wattle, blue gum trees and hakea; but gangs of labourers were still needed to shovel sand off the railway line that crossed the area. (4)

Constance was incensed by the plight of coloured people living on the Cape Flats in places like Windermere. They were regularly flooded out in low-lying areas during the winter months and suffered terribly from tuberculosis. On her charitable rounds, her pony and trap would be piled high with bread and cauldrons of homemade soup. Together with her husband she also ran a soup kitchen on a Saturday morning in Main Street, Plumstead, for the destitute.

She fumed, too, about the conduct of two property developers who bought up thousands of acres of land on the Cape Flats and then charged the host of squatters a high monthly rental for their smallholdings. The landowners provided nothing except standpipes for water, while making a mint of money in the process. This probably channelled her interests and abundant energy into becoming involved in politics.

Chapter 10
Suffragist and Town Councillor

In addition to her farming pursuits, Constance was deeply involved in the women's suffrage movement in Cape Town. By 1913 she had become a foundation member of the Alexandra Club and treasurer of the Women's Unionist Society. The suffragist movement spawned a proliferation of women's organisations dedicated to furthering their political influence and showing their competence in the political sphere. The term suffragette was only used to describe those who were involved in violent protest and the Cape scene was more sedate. With white, middle-class, English-speaking women as the driving force behind suffrage movements in South Africa, their interests tended to be circumscribed by their British imperialistic inheritance. This resulted in the exclusion of other female constituencies of class and colour. (1) But while their organisations might have been elitist and racist in representation, they still experienced sexual discrimination politically.

When the Union of South Africa was formed in 1910, women had to be satisfied with a supportive political role. Even so, the Women's Unionist Society was a powerful and articulate support group for the Unionist Party, which provided the official opposition in the first Union House of Assembly. Without the vote the women still made sure that their voices were heard in influential quarters and were a force to be reckoned with in challenging the *status quo*.

Having won the election, General Louis Botha and his followers had joined forces with other groups to found the South African Party. After the bitter legacy of the Anglo-Boer War (1899-1902), they were committed to the reconciliation of Boer and Briton. However, the SAP split when General Barry Hertzog and his supporters hived off and formed the National Party in 1915. They represented a radical Afrikaner nationalism, the divisive issue being their resistance to retaining close links with Britain. (2)

In contrast, the Unionist Party was imperialistic in its outlook, identifying with the English middle class in South Africa and wishing to maintain the closest possible ties with the Mother country. Commonly known as the 'Magnates' Party', it aimed to protect mining and commercial interests in South Africa against foreign competition. The main threat was cheap labour from India. This new Party came into being prior to Union following the merger of the pro-British, conservative Unionist Party of the Cape Colony with the Constitutional Party of the Free State. The Unionists were led by Dr. Leander Starr Jameson of the ill-fated Jameson Raid in December 1895, when he had headed an abortive attempt to overthrow President Paul Kruger of the Transvaal Republic. Not surprisingly, the founding members of the Unionists had mostly supported Britain in the subsequent hostilities.

The Women Unionists were a feisty group, not afraid to campaign on contentious issues. These included 'Hygiene' (a euphemism for sex education in schools), the Temperance Movement and the evils of drink, ignorance leading to the spread of disease, inadequate 'native' housing, and, after the outbreak of war in 1914, the support of Britain with war work. Lady Florence Phillips, wife of one of the wealthiest mining magnates in Johannesburg and Unionist Member of Parliament for Yeoville, was their outspoken leader and was known for her trenchant criticism of those in power. At one of the Women's meetings in her Johannesburg home, Florrie Phillips, as she was known, exhorted her followers to become actively involved in addressing fundamental social problems and in mounting an education campaign.

Farming was another of Florrie's passions and she took a leading role in running the vast estates owned by her husband, Sir Lionel Phillips, in the Northern Transvaal. She did not hesitate to upbraid the Government for failing to encourage agricultural development and for not attracting more English settlers to South Africa. In 1913, the Congress of Women Unionists elected her as president. Her rallying call to the members was to work for their country and for the Empire – for which their Government was doing so little. (3) Florrie regularly passed through Cape Town on her way overseas, so that Constance Wood's position as Treasurer of the Cape branch of the Society would bring them together. Florrie's role in founding the Women's Municipal Association in Johannesburg was another shared interest, as was the breeding of Jersey cows later on.

In 1920, a group of five hundred women from all over the country marched in procession up Government Avenue in Cape Town to place their demands for enfranchisement before the recently elected Prime Minister, General J.C. Smuts. Their petition had been signed by 54,500 women and the demonstration was led by a formidable array of female public figures. The select deputation that met with Smuts included a good number of titled ladies many of whom would not normally have concerned themselves with such affairs. Constance was part of this social circle as well as being deeply involved in the movement. Smuts offered them a vague promise of future legislation, but they had to wait another decade before they finally got the vote, and then it was for white women only.

As the opposition in Parliament, the Unionists often made life difficult for General Botha's Government. Their Party finally agreed to dissolve in 1921 when they were persuaded to merge with their adversaries, now led by General Smuts. In the face of mounting Nationalist opposition to remaining within the British Empire, the most pressing need for the white electorate was to strengthen the South African Party majority so as to keep it in power. (4) In 1934, the SAP-UP coalition finally came together to form the United Party. The economic hardships of the Great Depression had become a deciding factor in establishing a coalition government.

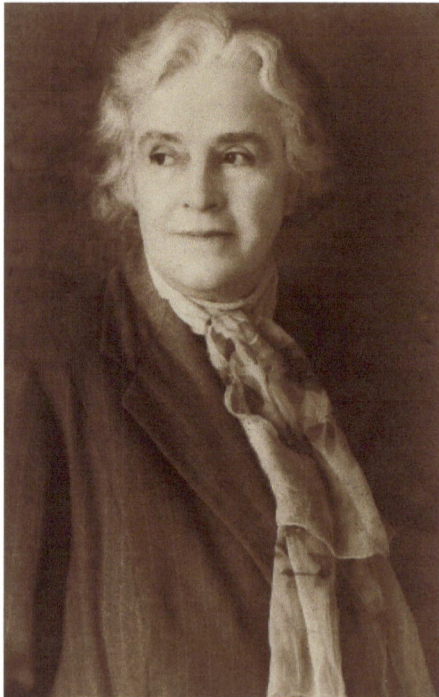

Throughout all these ups and downs, Constance retained a close interest in political affairs and did not hesitate to make her opinions heard. Murray Bisset, one of the Woods' near neighbours in Southfield Road and a well-known attorney and Test cricket captain, had become a Member of Parliament. When he put forward a Private Member's Bill that would allow first cousins to marry, Constance called it 'the Rabbit Act' and bombarded local newspapers with letters of denunciation. She also remained

Constance Clara Wood at 'Gledsmuir' (21)

56

fiercely loyal to the British Crown. Whenever the National Anthem was played, even over the radio in her own home, she would stand to attention. All other family members and staff were expected to do likewise, and they would remain standing until the Anthem was finished. We were brought up to follow the same routine.

On the more feminist front, the Alexandra Club was established by middle-class women in Cape Town as a move towards claiming social equality with men. Their club was the female equivalent of the City and Civil Service Clubs, a bastion of male dominance and power in British society that had been exported wholesale to the colonies. Inevitably, the women's egalitarian aspirations were the butt of cartoonists in the conservative press. (5) As a founding member of the Club, Constance's suffragist sympathies were abundantly clear. This was reinforced when the opportunity came for her to take the plunge and become actively involved in local government, causing a sensation and much tongue wagging among friends and neighbours.

In 1912 a municipal ordinance gave women who were property owners the right to vote alongside men in municipal elections, even though they were still excluded from becoming council members themselves. Only after the First World War did they finally gain this privilege. In the meantime, the formation of Union in 1910 had set in motion a process of unification that had filtered down to the municipal level. In 1913 the suburban municipalities stretching as far as Fish Hoek, and including Maitland, joined to form a single municipality with Cape Town. Wynberg alone, of which Plumstead was a part, resisted being incorporated into the wider whole. Water, or the lack of it, was a defining political issue for the other municipalities as they were dependent on the mother city for their water supply. A critical water shortage during the summer of 1913 had forced them to come together. (6)

With the approach of municipal elections in 1921, Wynberg was still clinging to its independence. The municipality's determination to hold on to its historic identity was partly due to its role as a longstanding service centre to the British garrison on Wynberg Hill. A more recent evolution, however, was the relationship between the business and professional interests of the old guard, who held the reins, and the rapidly expanding urban and commercial developments in the area. Large property owners were a significant force in resisting change, fearing a loss of the power and privilege associated with their position as wealthy merchants in the community. (7) One radical change they could not prevent was the opening up of municipal council membership to women. Thus it was that in September 1921, 'the notorious Mrs. C.C. Wood' achieved the distinction of being elected to the Wynberg Town Council. As such, she became one of the first two women town councillors in the Cape. The other was Mrs. Miriam Walsh in the Cape Town municipality.

Prior to the municipal election Constance had hung a big sign on her front gate: 'Vote for Constance Clara Wood'. On election day, Harry was packed off in a hansom cab to canvas from door to door accompanied by a school friend, Fred Searle, son of Judge Searle. Constance's slogan was 'Wake Up Wynberg'. She had obviously had enough of the conservative old guard even though many were neighbours or family friends. With their vested interests, they had held sway for decades putting a break on any modernising progress.

After Mr. Duncan Taylor had resigned, Constance stood against Dr. W.H. Rail of Diep River. As the wife of a much respected eye surgeon, she secured a large vote and came top of the polls. Not only was she the first woman on the council but she was also the first representative from the new residential area along Southfield Road. (8) Once on the council, however, although there were major changes in its policies, they put her in charge of the graves' department. This was hardly a wake-up call for Wynberg and she was very frustrated at having so little to do. The only positive outcome was in obtaining a huge slab of stone. This was used as a bridge over the small river at my home, Jersey Farm, Retreat. Dr. Rail went on to chair the newly-formed Southern Civic Association.

In the end Wynberg had to give in to unification with Cape Town. An insufficient water supply and an obsolete drainage system were contributory factors. But its largely residential character also played a significant part in its undoing. Without industrial development the municipality lacked sufficient economic resources to enable it to remain a viable independent entity. Wynberg was finally absorbed into the Greater Cape Town municipality in 1927, and the local council disbanded. (9)

Chapter 11
Jersey Cows, Ghosts, and the *Gita*

Family members have said how spooky they found 'Gledsmuir' with shutters banging in bedrooms even when there was no wind. One night the whole house was woken by the sound of the grandfather clock coming crashing down in the passage. They all rushed out in their nightclothes only to find the clock still standing upright, ticking steadily away. Constance herself seems to have had an interest in spiritualism. Together with her women friends they would play planchette. They believed that spirit messages would be written on a piece of paper when one of them rested their fingers lightly on a pencil. She may even have been psychic as she maintained that she could experience the presence of ghosts.

After her term of office as a municipal councillor was over, Constance devoted most of her time to farming, more especially dairying and cattle breeding. Harry remembered taking her to lunch with Sir Lionel and Lady Phillips in their home, Vergelegen, at the foot of the Hottentots Holland mountains in Somerset West. They now had a common interest in pedigreed Jersey cattle. On this occasion, however, Constance created something of a drama with her sensitivity to the supernatural.

The Phillips had recently retired to Vergelegen, the home of Willem Adriaan van der Stel, Governor at the Cape two hundred years previously. By the late 1910s the historic wine estate had become severely run down and it took five years and a good deal of the Phillips' money to restore the buildings and rehabilitate the farm. They were encouraged by the example of J.W. Jagger, a wealthy merchant and leader of the Unionist Party at the Cape, who had done much to develop Lourensford Estate next door.

At Vergelegen, Florrie started off by importing the first miniature Kerrie and Dexter cattle, but these were not a success. Then in 1922 she sunk even more of Sir Lionel's fortune into importing a substantial herd of pedigreed Jersey cattle from Jersey Island. Genetically this is one of the purest modern dairy breeds. Over hundreds of years, restrictive import legislation into the island and selective line breeding had maintained the highest quality of stock. (1) Florrie bought only the best animals, with record-breaking milk production, and was soon winning prizes at the annual Rosebank Show. By the 1930s the Vergelegen Jerseys had become a leading pedigreed herd, supplying cows and bulls to breeders throughout the country. Strangely enough some of the earliest Jersey breeders at the Cape were women. They included Mrs. Tracey of Vredenburg at Firgrove, Mrs. English of Lanzerac, Stellenbosch, and of

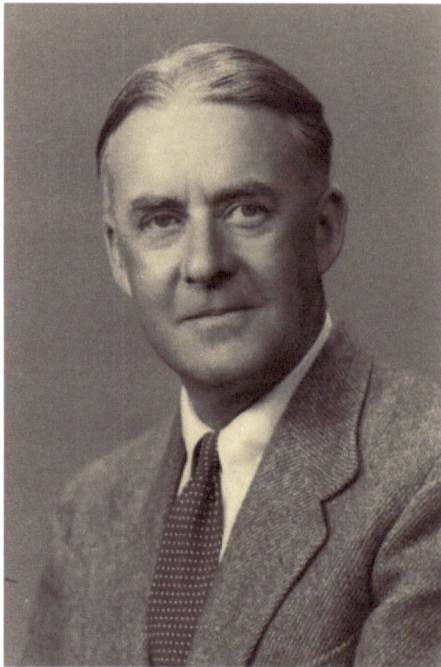

Harry Wood (22)

course Mrs. Constance Wood of Plumstead, who had been farming with them since 1916.

Florrie Phillips was renowned for her sumptuous luncheons at Vergelegen, not to mention her uninhibited remarks at table. She regularly hosted visiting dignitaries to the Cape including royalty. When Constance visited the historic homestead with my father she never got further than the front door. Much to Harry's embarrassment, his mother refused to enter the house claiming that there were too many ghosts around. Her meal had to be served to her on the stoep. Tom Barlow, who lived there many years later, claimed to have heard heavy footsteps echoing down the passages at night on a number of occasions.

After leaving school in 1924, Harry spent the next two years studying farming at Elsenburg College of Agriculture outside Stellenbosch. Founded in 1898, the College was the first of its kind in the country. It had recently amalgamated with the University of Stellenbosch to offer a new two-year diploma course in agriculture. During Harry's second year, his mother was one of the moving spirits who organised a meeting in the old lecture hall to form the Western Province Jersey Cattle Club. This was later called the Cape Jersey Cattle Club. Sir Lionel Phillips was elected chairman, with Sir Alec Versfeld and Mrs. Constance Wood as alternate Vice Chairmen. Mr. J.J. Roussouw and Harry were the other two founding members.

Jerseys are first thought to have been imported into South Africa in 1881, and the breed was initially confined to the Western Province. In 1905 the Stud Book Association was formed to encourage the stud breeding and registration of cattle, sheep, and all other domestic animals. The W.P Jersey Cattle Club was an offshoot of the mother body, the Jersey Breeder's Society of South Africa, which had been formed at a meeting in Pietermaritzburg in November 1920. Although Mrs. Constance Wood was one of the fourteen founding members, she much regretted that she was unable to attend and sent good wishes for the success of the new Society.

Sir Lionel Phillips was a good choice as chairman of the Cape branch of the Jersey breeders. With his substantial farming interests up north he had revived the Witwatersrand Agricultural Society and served as its president. He later became president of the Western Province Agricultural Society and immediately set about rebuilding and extending the Rosebank Show Grounds. These grounds were originally the site of the Zorgvliet vineyards, one of the first to be planted at the Cape. But after the vines died of phylloxera, the land was sold to Cecil John Rhodes. In 1894, he handed the property over to the Western Province Agricultural Society to be used for their annual show.

Although Florrie remained enthusiastic about her Jersey cattle, her poor health required frequent trips overseas to seek medical advice. She was also very involved in raising support for public art collections, and in helping to preserve historic Cape artefacts. But each year she still sent trainloads of prize-winning animals from Somerset West to the Rosebank Show. Meetings of the W.P. Jersey Cattle Club were held in the old wine cellar at Vergelegen, now restored as a library filled with antiques, followed by lunch. Harry would attend with his mother and during this time the Phillips invited him to come and manage the Vergelegen Jersey herd. He turned down the offer preferring to run his own dairy and breed his own stock.

By then Constance had acquired about twenty-five acres of land along Prince George Drive, on the road between Plumstead and Muizenberg, to provide more grazing for her cows. This became known as Jersey Farm, Retreat, and was not far from the sea. After leaving Elsenburg, Harry became farm manager and ran the dairy there until 1949. Initially, he lived in a large tin house, but on marrying Norah Hill, daughter of George Hill of Hill and Everett Importers, he built a double-storied thatched home. Situated in the midst of sand dunes on the Cape Flats, he created a beautiful garden with tree-lined pastures for the cows. This is where I was born and spent my childhood.

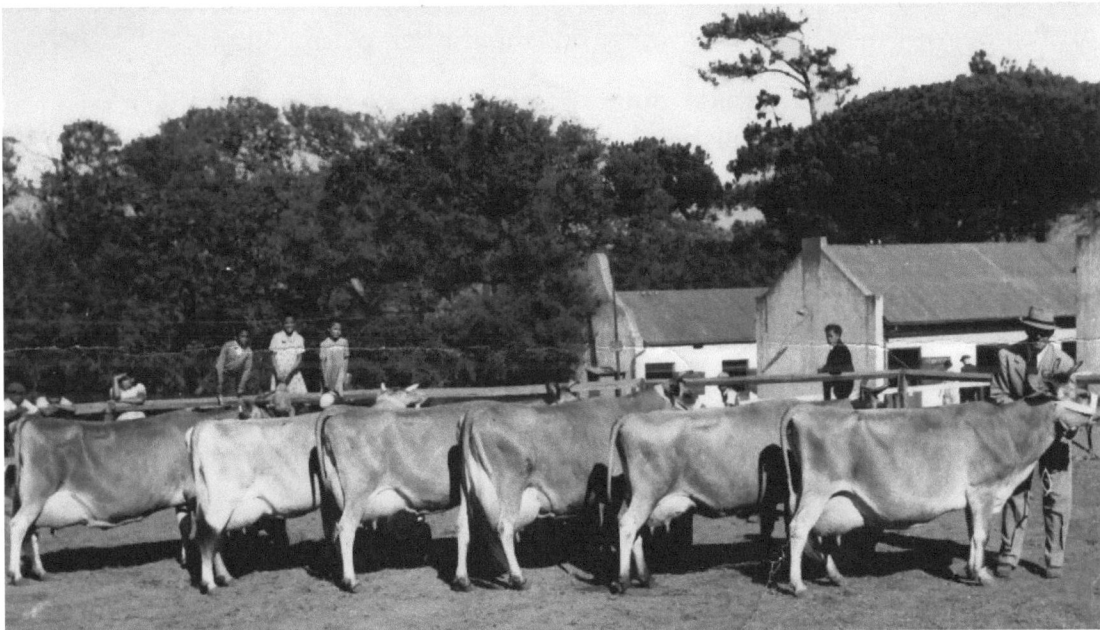

Harry Wood's prize-winning Jersey cows at Rosebank Show, 1952 (23)

Jersey farm was close to Princess Vlei, an oval basin fed by the Diep River. The vlei was popular with carp fishermen; and also sported pelicans, flamingos and many other water birds. White-flowered wateruintjies grew in profusion along the marshy edges. Wading into the water we would gather bucketfuls of the plant. They could be stewed in a mutton 'bredie', or else the bulbs were roasted, tasting like chestnuts. During the Cape winter the area would be plagued by floods. Work-seekers who had moved in as squatters in the sand dunes suffered greatly. In the early 1940s this led to the founding of the Cape Flats Distress Association by the formidable Miss Mary Attlee, sister of the future British Prime Minister. CAFDA was right opposite our farm and as children we would bicycle across Prince George Drive to help pack parcels of food and clothing to be given to destitute people.

In 1928 Harry, together with Alec Versfeld, was elected to the Jersey Council, and he remained a member for sixty-five years. In the forties he became the fifth president, and was later made an Honorary Life President. This was in recognition of his many years service as a senior judge of Jersey cattle in South Africa and Rhodesia, and of his prowess in building up the Gledsmuir herd. 'Gledsmuir' was used as his stud name. He had imported additional stock from Jersey Island and their progeny were regular prize-winners at Rosebank.

When my father moved to De Hoop farm in Bredasdorp, now enlarged as a Nature Conservation Reserve, he started experimenting with breeding hybrid proteas and exporting local *fynbos* and proteas overseas. This led to him becoming a founding member of the South African Protea Growers Association and to his editing their journal for some years. He had the same gift with words, the same sense of humour, and the same visionary imagination, as had his father before him.

Constance's intellect and wide range of interests was matched by her fondness for travel. At the time of her husband's death in 1937 she was on holiday in Mauritius. On a second visit the following year, she became friends with a Scottish Presbyterian minister, the Rev. John R. de Lingen. He was a poet, writer, linguist, classicist, philosopher, social reformer, and an authority on Indian culture. He had settled in Mauritius and his first book, published there in 1937, was called *The Golden Threshold: An Introduction to the Hindu Faith*. An annotated verse translation of *The Bhagavad Gita* from Sanskrit followed. Although not well known, it is regarded by a Sanskrit scholar as exceptional, as is De Lingen's understanding of Indian philosophy. (2) We have a copy of the *Gita* given to Constance shortly after its publication. It is inscribed by the author, 'To a dear friend, Mrs. Constance Wood, with the translator's warmest wishes', and is dated 26.viii.1938.

De Lingen and Constance were kindred spirits with many shared interests. With her fierce sense of solidarity with the oppressed members of the South African society, be they women, coloured and black people, or elderly men in straitened circumstance, she could identify with De Lingen's passion for justice for the beleaguered Indian community in Mauritius. He had been a founding member of the Indian Cultural Association. The ICA's goal was to galvanize the descendants of Indian migrants, who had replaced slaves as sugar-cane workers, into preserving their cultural identity and heritage, as well as fighting for racial equality under British imperialist rule. The *Gita* is a call to action in a world full of strife and injustice, so it is no wonder that De Lingen presented Constance with a copy of this ancient Hindu scripture.

Constance left 'Gledsmuir' after her husband's death and spent her remaining years at 'Umtali', in Ascot Road near Kenilworth Race Course. As a child I remember being extremely nervous of this grand old lady, who became ever more forceful with age. I was even more scared of her huge Great Danes who never left her side. They had been quite capable of leaping over the hefty front gates at 'Gledsmuir', a mere five feet high. One bitch regularly produced litters of up to sixteen puppies in a kaleidoscope of colours and would bite any intruder while caring for them. Constance Wood died after a stroke on 13 August 1943, aged 72. Her funeral took place at Plumstead Cemetery, she being buried with her husband. (3) Sadly, 'Gledsmuir' was ultimately pulled down and the land sold to make way for suburban housing developments.

✧

PART 4: 'A SCIENTIFIC SAINT'

Chapter 12
Eye Doctor To All

As the first to specialise in ophthalmology in South Africa, it was not long before D.J.W. had built up a large private practice. For just over twenty years he worked single-handedly, from 9 o'clock in the morning until 6.30 at night, his consulting hours having to fit in with his surgery. He thrived on this exacting regime and his reputation as a skilled eye doctor soon spread across the country. Popular with his patients, they found in him 'a most gentle, sympathetic and humane man and friend'. Although he confined himself to his speciality, he was consulted by many people who came for advice as to who they should see about other ailments. After examining their eyes he would then suggest various possibilities.

Even those who disagreed with D.J.W.'s political opinions, especially his fervent loyalty to the British Empire, still respected his medical skills and his integrity. One such was Monsignor Colbert (Kolbe?), a Roman Catholic priest, who told a mutual friend that 'Wood is a scientific saint in knowledge, gentleness and generosity, but oh, what dreadful opinions the man has!' This was at the time of the Anglo-Boer War when opposing camps were sharply divided by their political opinions. Later on, the Monsignor went on 'a disappointing excursion' to Lourdes. On returning he confessed that everything Wood had told him had been fulfilled to the letter. He added that, 'I have the painful satisfaction of knowing that my doctor's opinion was right'. (1)

D.J.W. was fond of music and his children played the piano and violin. His baby grand piano is now in the possession of Geoff Montgomery in Smithfield. Geoff is a gifted pianist and organist who has accompanied worship in many different churches around South Africa and Zimbabwe. One of the Wood family's favourite outings was to be taken by train to Cape Town on a Thursday evening to attend a symphony concert in the City Hall. The Cape Town Municipal Orchestra had been formed in 1914 and D.J.W. had his own box overlooking the orchestra. The family must have attended the inaugural concert in February that year when the programme included the Overture to the Meistersingers of Wagner and the unfinished symphony of Schubert. The conductor was Theo Wendt. (2)

Monsieur Colbert would sit below the Wood family in the front row. Because of his poor eyesight he would study his programme with a torch an inch away from his eyes. After the priest had had a cataract operation, for which D.J.W. had gained renown, he looked up to their box and waved his programme to show how he could now read it on his knees. In those days cataract surgery was performed without stitches. After the operation the patient would have to lie still for up to ten days with sandbags holding his head in place. The thick spectacle lenses used to replace the diseased lens of the eye were unsightly and could distort vision, but at least the patient's sight had been restored. (3)

Dr. C.M. Murray, who joined his father's ophthalmic practice in 1904, was impressed by D.J.W.'s youthful appearance, wonderful vitality and sheer brilliance. On a personal level, Murray valued the eye surgeon's 'kindliness of manner and quiet sense of humour, which gained the confidence of his patients and endeared him to his friends'. When asked to examine the eyes of Murray's six-year old daughter, she told her father afterwards that 'Dr. Wood says my eyes are very good. Perhaps in about 40 years I might want some glasses, but if I wanted to see him then I had better bring a spade'. (4)

The moving testimony of another young patient was given my father in 1963. (5) Marguerita Herold, nee Rita Woolley, was then eighty-four years' old and was living in King William's Town. Her father, Paymaster Rear Admiral Charles Woolley, C.M.G., R.N. had been appointed to Simonstown at the turn of the century. They had been transferred from Malta, much to her South African mother's delight. As a cadet paymaster on a Royal Navy sailing ship, Charles Woolley had met his future wife, Julia Marian Marguerite van der Riet, on a previous visit to the naval base at the Cape. Julia's father was the Resident Magistrate and Civil Commissioner at Simonstown, and she was his 13th surviving child.

Around 1902, after Rita Woolley's family had settled into a cottage at Admiralty House, it was noticed that one of the six year old's eyes was developing a bad squint. She was taken to see Dr. Wood. He diagnosed her as suffering from 'glare stroke due to the brilliant blue sea in the Mediterranean and brighter sunlight upon it'. In Malta her English nanny had told her that babies loved the 'twinkles' on the water, so aggravating her condition. Rita remembered being scared of Dr. Wood's big chair and all the lights he used. But, as she said:

He understood and talked to me of my sailor suit, asking if children teased me for the eye that was 'all crooked'. He was a very clever psychiatrist and won my heart, so that when I had to face 'drops' that made everything look big, and find that I would need spectacles, I did not resent it. He told me that I could help him by wearing my glasses and trying not to break them. But often I had to go back for repair.

One dreadful day Rita's older brother Eric mounted her on their pony, bare backed and without a bridle. He then gave the animal a good whack on its stern. She went careering off, landing in the middle of a garden party in Admiralty House. Rita remembered being 'horribly untidy and without glasses'. Next day she was much mortified when her father took her to see Dr. Wood and told him how naughty she had been.

But Dr. Wood said he understood how embarrassing it was to be taken to a party like that, and even more humiliating to have to come and tell him I had lost his specs. He said he knew a little boy who needed small specs and Eric must go and find them in the grass so he could fix them; and he would give me a bigger pair because I was growing so fast I needed them.

When the Woolleys returned to England, Rita went to an eye specialist in Cambridge. During World War I, her eye problems left her working in the Forestry Corps, felling and cutting pit props for the muddy trenches. Over many years special lenses and daily exercises gradually drew the pupil of her eye into place and aided the recovery of her sight. Whenever she had her eyes examined, Dr. Wood's report went with her and at no stage was the treatment changed or brought more up to date. After her marriage to a South African soldier they were repatriated to the Cape. Having gained a higher maths qualification for Map Compilation, she was employed in Aircraft House. Her vision was now good enough to use a stereoscope and epidioscope. She ends her story saying: 'By this you will know how grateful I must always be to a very real friend, a clever, capable Eye Specialist, who made all the difference to my life. At 84 years I can still paint, read, and live normally. God bless those who are honouring the name of the man who has done so much for others.'

For a good many years D.J.W. also served as ophthalmologist to the Railway Medical Service. Steel splinters in their eyes were one of the many hazards suffered by train drivers and other railway workers. In 1928, word came that he was to be retired from this work prematurely but the Railway Medical Officers successfully petitioned the Minister of Railways and Harbours, the Hon. C.W. Malan. They said that:

Dr. Wood's reputation as an Eye Specialist is second to none in South Africa, and we feel that his retirement from the Service, at a time when his skill and judgment are at their zenith, will deprive the railwaymen and their families of a specialist of unusual character and skill, and the Railway Medical Officers of a Consultant in whom they have the completest confidence. (6)

Throughout his career D.J.W. gave his services to the poor of Cape Town free of charge. (7) One example was his work with children from the Athlone School for the Blind. This institution had been established by the Rev. Arthur Blaxall (1891-1970), the Anglican rector at Maitland, after he discovered that there was no schooling available for any blind children of colour. The only other such school in the Union was in Worcester, in the Cape Province, to which they were unable to obtain admission.

With the help of Walter Bowen, an advocate and politician who had lost his sight during World War I, and with the aid of a partial State subsidy, they managed to raise enough money to buy a small house for boarders and to pay the salary of a special teacher, Mrs. Lawrence. In May 1927, six apprehensive blind boys and girls were introduced to the Earl of Athlone, the Governor-General, when he opened the building and gave it his name. (8)

As word spread, African, Indian and coloured children started coming from all over the country, and the school rapidly outgrew its facilities. After more fund-raising the school was moved to Faure in 1931. The pupils were housed in wood-and-iron dormitories, which had originally been used on Robben Island but had since been dismantled and brought to the mainland. Arthur Blaxall served as superintendent at Faure from 1932 to 1937, while Walter Bowen remained chairman for twenty-one years. (9) In addition to standard pre-school and primary education, the pupils were taught Braille and music as well as being given vocational training. Run on Christian lines, the words: 'Thine Eyes Shall See The King In His Beauty' stood over the entrance to the open-air chapel. (10)

Blaxall recalls that on admission every new boarder was taken to see Dr. D.J. Wood – 'the eye specialist whose name is known far and wide beyond the circle of Cape Town'. Several pupils had a measure of their sight restored by surgical treatment. In 1933 a rural Venda boy, Romboho, heard about the school and begged to be given a place. Desperate for education, he travelled alone by train to the Cape, ending the journey by donkey cart. Despite the boy's natural fear of doctors and hospitals he consented 'to be cut' by Dr. Wood.

The matron reported that when Romboho left hospital 'he stopped and just gazed at the new world in which forms and figures were now clearer and better defined than ever before'. He had to return to hospital for further operations, and was still technically blind, but he was 'greatly enriched by the added measure of sight. How precious is such a gift!' wrote Blaxall: 'Truly to doctors and surgeons it is sometimes given to be restorers of physical beauty, to lighten and gladden the lives of men. Such a gift must be carefully guarded, and jealously watched.' (11)

In 1935, a special class was started at the school for those children for whom some sight had been restored by surgical treatment. A different technique of education was followed, carefully planned, to prepare them for a probable return to ordinary sighted life. There would always be borderline cases, but the joke was that in the entire country the only special education offered to children with seriously defective vision was for those of colour. Indeed, quite a few were able to return home to work in the sighted world.

During the First World War, D.J.W. extended this humanitarian work to treating all soldiers and sailors with eye problems free of charge. Among the family papers is correspondence relating to the arrangements for his services. At the start, Louis Botha, Minister for Defence, approved his being placed on the Reserve of Officers with the rank of Major. He was officially appointed Honorary Ophthalmic Surgeon at No.1 General Hospital in Wynberg. A Government car fetched him at Wynberg station for his weekly visit, or else he would catch a taxi. He was also allowed to see some military patients in his consulting rooms in Cape Town, and serious surgical cases were admitted to the New Somerset Hospital.

After the war, grateful thanks for his patriotic assistance came from Louis Botha himself, as well as the Brigadier General of the South African Military Command at the Castle in Cape Town, the Vice Admiral in Chief at Simonstown, and the Lords Commissioners of the Admiralty in London. He was told that had he not undertaken this work they would have had to withdraw vitally needed medical officers from the field of operations. (12)

Chapter 13
Surgeon, Teacher and Clinician

In 1896, D.J.W. was appointed part-time Honorary Ophthalmic Surgeon to the New Somerset Hospital and started a weekly Eye Clinic. In 1913 he was appointed as First Specialist. Opened in 1862, the double storey hospital building, with its turreted corners, looked more like a modest castle than a hospital. (1) Sir George Grey, Governor at the Cape, had laid the cornerstone three years earlier and chosen the Tudor style of the building. The original hospital in Chiappini Street was named after Lord Charles Somerset, a previous Governor, who had given land for its construction. The new building was situated in Green Point between the Chavonnes Battery (now the Clocktower in the docks) and the town.

Additions and extensions were added to the hospital over the years, the number of beds more than doubled, and a new operating theatre installed. None the less, when the University of Cape Town became associated with the hospital in 1917, it was woefully overcrowded, ill equipped, and antiquated. It was hardly ideal as a teaching hospital for medical students.

Thanks to generous benefactors, the 'Shipley Pavilion' was opened in August 1916 to accommodate the first ophthalmic and aural diseases (Ear, Nose and Throat) Departments. (2) With its four wards of eight beds each, new outpatient facilities and more modern equipment, conditions were decidedly better than in the main building. According to Dr. J. Luckoff, the Honorary E.N.T. Surgeon at Somerset Hospital, 'the partnership proved harmonious and created a valuable hospital unit of separate twins'. (3)

As a surgeon, D.J.W. was strict and the nurses were said to be terrified of him; but meticulous post-operative care was vital to the success of his surgery. He was supported by the dedication and dynamic efficiency of the sister in charge, Sister Mott. A highly qualified nurse, she had received special Ophthalmic training at Moorfields Eye Hospital, and was credited with creating 'the order and the spirit' of Shipley Pavilion. History relates that the department gained an excellent reputation 'under the guidance of the eminent ophthalmologist, Dr. D.J. Wood'. (4)

For all his kindly disposition, D.J.W. remained suspicious of each new Oculist. In the end he accepted them and they worked together, albeit rather reluctantly. Thursday was 'Eye' day when he saw outpatients in the morning and operated in the afternoon. According to Professor Justin van Selm, he was particularly well known for his work on the histology of scleritis, having enucleated both eyes from a patient who had the condition and who demanded the operations because of the intractable pain. (5)

D.J.W. continued on his own at the hospital until 1919 when Dr. S.J. du Toit was appointed temporarily as Assistant Surgeon. Du Toit had started practising as the second ophthalmologist in Cape Town three years earlier, relieving his colleague of some of the pressure. But he had to wait another decade before he was promoted permanently as Assistant Surgeon. Dr. A.W.S. Sichel joined him the following year and Dr. F.B. Dreyer became the third registrar. (6)

The University of the Cape of Good Hope was established in Cape Town in 1873. This was only an examining body and students took their courses through post-matriculation studies at the South African College in association with the Diocesan College. Starting in 1904, these schools gradually developed a three-year course covering a range of medical subjects. Finally, an Act was passed in 1916 creating the University of Cape Town and it was formally established two years later. When UCT opened a medical faculty in 1916, D.J.W. was one of the first to offer his services. Beginning as an Honorary Visiting Ophthalmic Surgeon, he was made Lecturer in Ophthalmology in 1919. The Faculty only became fully fledged in 1920 when it appointed its first clinical professors, making it the oldest medical school in Southern Africa. D.J.W. was also a member of the Advisory Committee to the Faculty Board.

The regulations and curriculum for the degrees of M.B., Ch.B. were introduced in 1928, but teaching remained limited to undergraduates until 1950. The ophthalmology course consisted of a weekly formal lecture followed by demonstrations in the outpatient clinic. The course lasted two years and ended with an examination. Classes were given to sixth year students during the first two quarters, while the clinical work took place on Thursdays at the hospital. D.J.W. remained head of the Department of Ophthalmology until his death. As one of the pioneers in establishing the medical school, his outstanding work was said to have brought honour to the University. (7) In the 1930s the number of medical students doubled necessitating an increase in staff and an expansion of the curriculum, especially in clinical work.

The many facets of D.J.W.'s work gave him a unique opportunity of combining his clinical cases with original research in his laboratory, hence his extensive collection of mounted pathology specimens, sections, models, photographs, demonstration drawings and paintings. Added to this was the wealth of notes, scientific papers and addresses at meetings, which were published in medical journals at home and abroad over more than forty years. His international reputation was recognised by *The British Journal of Ophthalmology* in 1917 when he was appointed the first South African

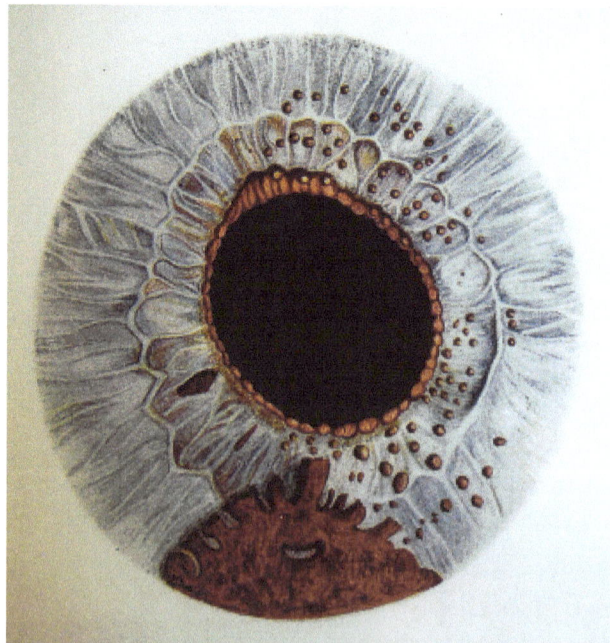

Slit-lamp painting by D.J.W. - 'Melanosis of
the Iris and New Formation of a Hyaline
Membrane on its Surface', *BJO XII* 1928 .
Opthalmology Department,
Groote Schuur(24)

representative on their editorial board, and this lasted until his death. (See Appendix 2 and 3 for a list of his publications).

D.J.W. was ever alert to new developments in ophthalmology and was always keen to share his knowledge with colleagues, as much in practical demonstrations as in print. So, for example, there is a brief report in the *South African Medical Record (SAMR)* of a scientific and social evening at UCT in which he demonstrated the use of the new Slit-Lamp and Corneal Microscope. The slit-lamp, used in conjunction with a biomicroscope, was developed by Alvar Gullstrand in 1911. Although it was a major breakthrough in facilitating a detailed examination of both the anterior and posterior segments of the eye for diagnostic and therapeutic purposes, it was some time before it became widely used. (8) The binocular slit-lamp examination provides a stereoscopic magnified view of the eye structures, and is now commonly used to detect a variety of eye conditions. These include corneal injury, conjunctivitis, retinal detachment, retinitis pigmentosa, macular degeneration, and much else. (9)

In D.J.W.'s time a course of post-graduate training had yet to be established. The general rule for aspiring ophthalmologists was to begin with six to twelve months as a house surgeon in the Eye Department. They would then be allowed to attend the outpatient department for about a year as honorary clinical assistants. After that they would have to go overseas for six to twelve months to attend specialised lectures and clinics, mainly at Moorfields Eye Hospital. Finally, they would write an examination for the Diploma in Ophthalmic Medicine and Surgery (D.O.M.S.) of London, Dublin or elsewhere. In 1933, Dr. K. Cunningham was the first Cape Town graduate to work as house surgeon under D.J.W. in Shipley Ward before going abroad to finish his training. Once a new system of paid full-time and part-time posts was instituted in 1951, it became possible for post-graduates to complete their specialist training at Groote Schuur. (10)

D.J.W. continued with his undergraduate teaching until a few weeks before his death. Then, to his intense disappointment, failing health compelled him to resign. A few days before the commencement of the new term he handed his lecture notes to Dr. J.S. du Toit, who was now on the staff at UCT, saying, 'Take them with my blessing. I hope you will find them of some use after the blue pencil has been used liberally'.

Du Toit was one of many who testified to D.J.W.'s devotion to his work, for it had been the most absorbing interest of his life, both in private practice and in hospital surgery. Even when D.J.W.'s health was failing he had continued to work full time, and had done his quota of operations at the eye hospital a week before his death. Du Toit praised him for being 'a keen and energetic clinician in every detail, with a full measure of the untiring patience which ophthalmology demands, and unwilling to pass his responsibilities to others'. (11)

During his last years, D.J.W. took a lively interest in the construction of Groote Schuur Hospital. The outlay and equipment of the eye department were of special concern and he eagerly anticipated working with better facilities. It was not to be for he died before the hospital was finished in 1938. On completion, the ophthalmic staff at New Somerset moved to Groote Schuur to start the new Eye Department. Through bold planning and personal clout, D.J.W. and Dr. J. Luckoff had insisted on more space for their new Eye and E.N.T. Departments than was deemed necessary at the time. In the eye section this allowed generous accommodation for an Optician, Orthoptist, retinal camera, tonometry room, septic theatre and light coagulator room. Before long other departments gradually sneaked their way in, the cardiac clinic being the chief invader, leaving the ophthalmic host with restricted movement and growth.

The Eye Department started out with fifty beds in the north-west wing of the new hospital, divided equally between people of different racial origin. With a dramatic increase of outpatients over the years, the number of eye clinics had to be increased. Dr. Townsend recalled that under apartheid, racial segregation in the clinics was achieved by having people of different colour sit back to back in rows. (12)

Following D.J.W.'s death, Dr. Alan W.S. Sichel and Dr. J.S. du Toit were appointed jointly as Senior Surgeons to the Eye Department and as lecturers in ophthalmology, while still heading their own Firms. They went on to hold many prestigious positions in the medical field before they retired at the end of 1950. Both were awarded the Gold Medal of the Medical Association of South Africa for distinguished services to their profession. (13)

In 1938, Dr. Leonard Townsend took over D.J.W.'s practice in Cape Town, in the same rooms off Church Square with the same homemade furniture. A Rhodesian by birth, Townsend had trained as an eye surgeon at the Royal Westminster Ophthalmic Hospital in London. He had then built up a thriving practice in Bulawayo before coming to the Cape. Here he was appointed Assistant Clinical Lecturer in Ophthalmology at UCT and an honorary staff member of the Shipley Pavilion. After the outbreak of World War II he joined the South African Medical Corps and served in the rank of Major in East Africa and the Middle East. On his return, he resumed his private practice as well as becoming Head of Ophthalmology and Senior Lecturer at the University. In 1961 he resigned through ill health; but continued as head of his Firm for a while longer. He remembered D.J.W. as being 'a shy, refined, aesthetic man keen on scientific advancement'. (14)

Chapter 14
Blind Lepers on Robben Island

Yet another of D.J.W.'s posts was as Ophthalmic Surgeon to the Robben Island Leper Institution. The 'Island of Seals' had long been used as a penal settlement and dumping ground for political exiles. Its location at the entrance to Table Bay, five miles from Cape Town, ensured that those who were thought to be dangerous to the social order were kept well out of reach and unable to escape. In 1846 the Colonial Government finally closed the prison and replaced it with a hospital for chronically sick poor people, lepers and 'lunatics'.

In 1817, Moravian missionaries had established the first leper colony in the country in the Hemel-en-Aarde (Heaven and Earth) valley, between Hermanus and Caledon. This lasted until 1845 when the lepers were removed to Robben Island. At first they were confined to their settlement on a voluntary basis and were free to leave if they wished. This changed after the Leprosy Suppression Act was passed in May 1892. At that time there was no cure for leprosy, and the manner in which the disease was spread was unknown. With a growing fear that the so-called 'black peril' was contagious, the public wanted the lepers off the mainland and out of sight. This xenophobia led to their compulsory detention, which was legally enforced.

For many years most of the leper patients were black, destitute, mostly male and in the advanced stage of the disease. Their geographical isolation was supposed to prevent them from contaminating others. (1) After the Act was passed, admission was no longer voluntary and their movement was restricted. Before then an average of twenty-five lepers had been admitted to Robben Island a year. In 1892 this rose to 338, and in 1893 a further 250 were admitted. (2) Some were tricked into going thinking that after a few months treatment they would be released home, only to find that it was a life sentence. Others were taken away from their families in handcuffs. (3)

In the beginning the lepers lived in appalling conditions. They were wretchedly housed in old chicken coops or 'pondoks', were badly fed and had little or no medical treatment. They felt like prisoners and at one stage burnt down their dwellings in protest in order to get better housing. Their rebellion was largely unsuccessful and leper police were brought in to control them. A minor reform was the giving of free passes to visiting families. (4) But many relatives feared crossing the sea in a small boat and the Island was often cut off by bad weather. A visiting physician in 1881 reported: 'Here I saw human beings kennelled worse than dogs. In a long, low, thatched shed some forty poor creatures were stowed away, most of them unable to leave their beds. Here were black, half-caste and white all mixed together, but no females'. (5) An educated man such as a schoolmaster would have been dumped among illiterates.

Leprosy has been known since biblical times, with any skin disease being thought to be a curse from sinful behaviour. In 1893 Dr. Armauer Hansen, a Norwegian, discovered that it was caused by a bacterium – *Myobacterium leprae*. It became known as Hansen's disease and was now considered treatable if not curable. If left untreated it is most likely to be spread by coughing or sneezing, but most people have a natural immunity.

The earliest sign is usually a spot of a different colour on the skin. This may become numb with loss of hair and lead to disfiguring skin lesions. The leprosy bacteria affect the nerves in hands and feet leading to sensory loss in the extremities and muscular weakness. The long-term result is infections in the injured areas and permanent damage. Fingers and toes may be lost, and feet might have to be amputated. In the nose, scarring in the internal lining may lead to its collapse. The eyes are particularly sensitive as the bacteria attack the nerves surrounding them causing the loss of the blinking reflex. Blinking moistens the eye and protects it from injury such as scratches or debris. The numbness of the eye and other severe complications may eventually lead to blindness. (6) Leprosy has two common forms, tuberculoid and lepromatous, the latter being the most severe with large disfiguring nodules.

Robben Island was a sandy, treeless waste, and extremely unhealthy for sick people. The mornings were invariably foggy or misty, the days hot, while a cold wind blew in the evenings. The glare from sun and sea were disastrous for the lepers' eyes, and the damp climate was equally bad for their weak chests. They were cared for by a small band of devoted nurses who would spend hours bandaging wounds, cleaning wards, and monitoring progress. (7) There were three chapels: St. Mary's for female lepers, the Good Shepherd for the men, and a Children's chapel. A number of All Saints sisters from England had the care of leper children, and the sisters' training in nursing and education was invaluable. (8)

During the day those who were mobile were allowed to roam much of the Island. Many found solace in fishing off the rocks. Others made small gardens and sold the produce to the officials. Some were given low wages working in the laundry, or as tailors, needlewomen, cooks, painters, plasterers, and sanitary workers. But they all had to be in bed by 10 p.m. (9) There were those who planned to escape by building boats. These would be broken up by officials before completion. Even so, the intrepid builders would start again.

When D.J.W. made his first inspection as Eye Surgeon in 1913, only 'lunatics' and lepers remained on the Island. The crossing was still daunting in a small steamer, which often had to brave rough weather in wind and rain. The vessel had to be boarded by jumping from the wooden jetty near the clock tower in Victoria Basin onto the deck, challenging for women with their long skirts. On arrival at the Island the steamer anchored in the bay. Officials and important passengers were taken by rowing boat to the jetty. The rest were bundled with the cargo into a longboat manned by convicts.

By then a commission had sat to listen to the lepers' grievances, and conditions had improved somewhat. At the time, though, despite the fact that the complainants were not infectious and only slightly contagious, guards had been placed between them and the commissioners, and the lepers had been forbidden to approach the table. (10) Soon afterwards a new block was built for male lepers with more satisfactory sanitary arrangements. White paying patients were housed separately leading to discriminatory treatment.

In his report on 'The Eye Complications of Leprosy', D.J.W. begins by saying: 'If loss of ability to work and to enjoy life, added to actual suffering, be a test of the importance of a disease, then the ocular manifestations of leprosy must be given a high place'. In all the varieties of leprosy he saw, the number suffering from eye disease was disproportionately high. In the anaesthetic form, the eyes and adnexa (accessory organs of the eye including the eyelids and lacrymal apparatus) were seriously affected in more than half the cases of those up to the age of sixty. He also noted desiccation of their exposed corneas together with ulcers and opacities. In the tubercular variety, the eyes were attacked directly by the disease and 90% became blind within the first decade. In the end, if they managed to survive the ravages of their disease, all were more or less blind.

Continuing his report, D.J.W. found that the most serious cause of loss of sight amongst the lepers was irido-cyclitis. The problem was that the condition began insidiously and was well developed before acute attacks were felt. Invariably it led to the occlusion of the pupil, opacity of the cornea, lens and vitreous, with the shrinking of the eyeball. D.J.W believed that some of his findings - such as the large numbers of minute yellow, rounded, raised points, scattered haphazardly over the iris in every case of irido-cyclitis, and not seen in other forms of iritis – were pathognomonic, and were being described for the first time.

He feared that the treatment of any of these eye problems was 'exceedingly hopeless' seeing that the primary disease was still incurable. In the anaesthetic form he thought that efficient protection of the eyes was the best means at their disposal. This included wearing goggles, cleanliness through frequent irrigation of saline solution or boric lotion, and the occasional use of a mild astringent. In conclusion, he is unsparing in his criticism of the deplorable living conditions of the lepers, and urged the importance of selecting a proper site for such a settlement:

We may not, in South Africa, find a place with cool streams, shady trees, and a mild and quiet atmosphere, but we need not, therefore, choose the most acute antithesis possible. It cannot be that an island where water supply is not only bad but hopelessly inadequate, where the roads are laden with dust, where a tree worthy of the name refuses to grow, and where the only shade is the galvanised iron verandah, is in any way the proper place to confine for life those whose visual troubles form one of their most serious and distressing disabilities. (11)

D.J.W. was deeply disturbed by his work with lepers though fascinated by his findings. In 1925, he returned to the subject of 'Ocular Leprosy' in a paper published in *The British Journal of Ophthalmology*. (12) In his article he states that 'one of the deepest tragedies in the life of the unfortunates who contract leprosy is the affection of sight, which occurs in some form or other in nearly all cases if they live long enough'.

By now he had a number of patients who were 'sufficiently presentable' to be permitted to come to the mainland, some weekly, to attend his clinic. There he could better study their diseased eyes with the latest equipment, such as a slit-lamp and binocular microscope, instead of the naked eye. One of them was a young Jewish boy of about twenty-one, who had contracted leprosy ten years previously. His right eye had had to be removed because of the pain and had been sent to Moorfields for further examination. The boy's other eye was in a pretty bad state too; but D.J.W. was excited by the thought that some new, and rather unusual treatment, was offering encouraging results, as described in his article.

After giving a precise account of the ravages of leprosy in the boy's diseased eye, he went on to describe his efforts to stem its customary advanced progression. Having failed to get any response using subconjunctival injections with bicyanide of mercury, he added some purified ox gall to his solution to increase the vulnerability of the bacilli. Later, he added 1% strength of pure sodium taurocholate. Almost from the start there was a marked improvement even though the patient, who was supposed to be a nearly arrested case, had a severe relapse affecting his arms and legs. D.J.W. well knew that in a slowly progressive disease such as leprosy, a year was not sufficient to build up more than hope, but with the cessation of the iritis and the disappearance of the more superficial ocular disease, the treatment had seemed very promising.

It was another six years before the leper colony on Robben Island was closed and moved to Westfort Hospital in Pretoria. (13) By then, leprosy had declined in the

Western Cape and the high cost of maintaining the institution with an all-white staff had become untenable. Moreover, the compulsory segregation of former times had given way to a more liberal isolation policy for infectious cases on the mainland. When the lepers finally left the Island all their buildings were destroyed.

In the meantime, Howard, D.J.W.'s eldest son, was for many years the doctor on the Island. In 1931, he moved with his leper patients to Westfort, ending up as Deputy Superintendent of the Hospital. Howard was the only doctor in the family but he struggled to follow in his father's illustrious footsteps. Unable to meet the high expectations of those around him he was saddled with an overwhelming inferiority complex. Alcohol was his undoing and he died a tragic death.

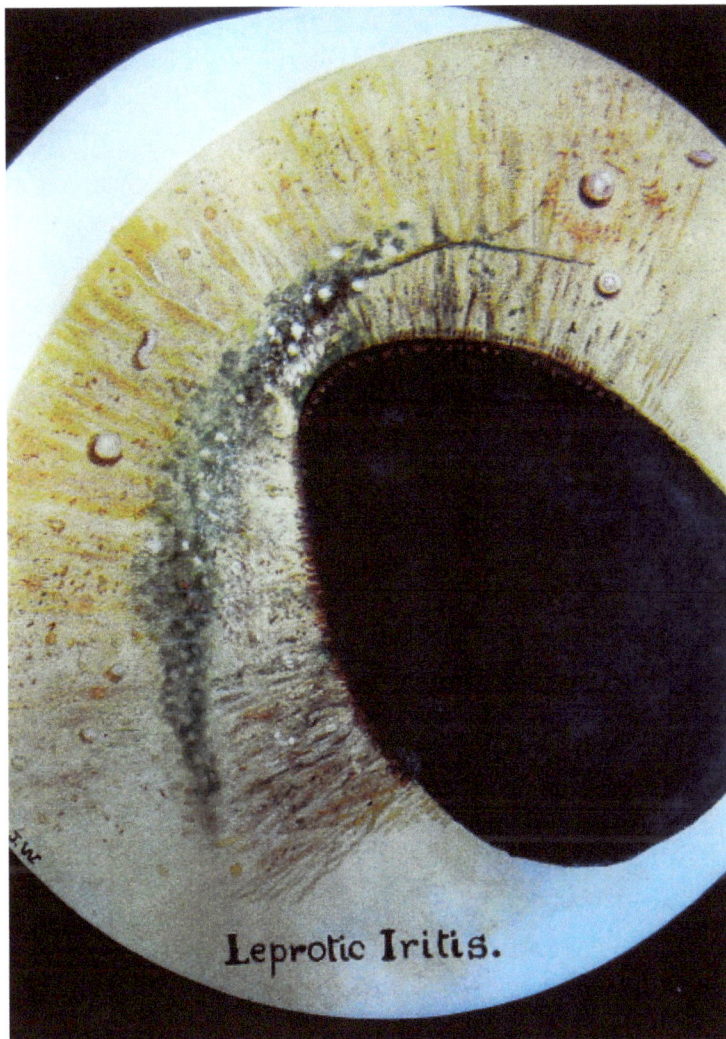

Slit-lamp painting of 'Leprotic Iritis'
by D.J.W., in BJO 1925 (25)

Chapter 15
Vaccines, District Surgeons and Dentistry

From the start of his career, D.J.W. was deeply interested in all that had to do with the organization and conduct of the medical profession as a whole, and was actively involved in a variety of governing bodies, helping to found some. Beginning with the British Medical Association (B.M.A.), he served as secretary of the local Cape of Good Hope (Western) Branch (CGH) in the 1890s and, later, as President. He was regarded as an indefatigable member, attending all its meetings, presenting papers, showing cases, and joining in discussions and debates. (1) The Branch's books were also kept in his surgery.

When the B.M.A. amalgamated with the Medical Association of South Africa in 1926, he was as enthusiastic a supporter of the new body as he had been of the old. Dr. C.M. Murray, whose father had been a friend and colleague, considered that 'no one was more deeply sensitive of the value to the profession of this link with the organizations of the Old Country'. At the start of his career, Murray had greatly appreciated the fact that at B.M.A. meetings D.J.W. had always been gentle and encouraging in his criticisms, and unfailingly sympathetic to younger members: 'He had the gift of drawing them out and spurring them to further efforts in the cause which he had so much at heart.' (2)

D.J.W. was not only interested in new developments in his own field, but read widely in different branches of the profession and kept abreast of advances in medicine and surgery in other countries. During his overseas leaves he lost no opportunity in attending post-graduate courses and visited various continental clinics, such as Vienna and Paris. (3) At the end of 1905, he went on one of his comparatively rare trips to England just about the time Sir Almroth Wright (1861-1947), the leading bacteriologist and immunologist in Britain, brought out his work on vaccines. Although this was quite outside D.J.W.'s field, he was fascinated with the new preventive medicine - based on biology, bacteriology, physiology, pathology and pharmacology. Consequently, he spent a good deal of his visit working with Wright in his research laboratory at St. Mary's Hospital Medical School in Paddington, London.

As professor of pathology, Wright had worked closely with the British armed forces in developing his vaccines, and was the first to develop a system of anti-typhoid (enteric) fever inoculation. This had been used successfully during the recent Anglo-Boer War. (4) However, too many soldiers still died from easily preventable diseases. When World War I broke out he convinced the armed forces to embark on an extensive programme of immunising the troops, saving many lives from infection.

During his time at St. Mary's, D.J.W. was kept busy doing laboratory work, studying the case notes of Wright's patients, and in seeing for himself their remarkable response to this groundbreaking treatment, especially with tubercular gland disease. For him, they were 'the greatest triumphs of therapeutic methods which have come under my notice'. (5) He even wondered if vaccine inoculations might not assist in the treatment of leprosy. On returning home he lost no time in sharing his enthusiasm and new expertise with the medical fraternity. Barnard Fuller observed that 'it was obvious that he had made a very thorough study of what was then a new and rather puzzling subject'. (6)

Early in 1906, D.J.W. used his inaugural address as President of the Cape Western Branch of the B.M.A., to present his audience with a barrage of information on 'The Treatment of Bacterial Diseases by Vaccines'. (7) Beginning with a brief resume of the pioneering studies of Jenner, Pasteur, Lister and Koch, D.J.W. went on to explain the value of the opsonic index, a key factor in Wright's work. Opsonin, derived from the Greek word *opsonion* meaning victuals or food provision, is an antibody developed in blood serum that causes bacteria or other foreign cells to become more susceptible to the action of phagocytes in the healing process. The opsonic index is the ratio of the amount of opsonin in the blood of a person with an infectious disease to that present in a healthy person. This provided an easy and certain way of obtaining information as to someone's state of immunity and of determining the appropriate dosage in injecting a vaccine during the inoculation process.

Not content with a mere overview of the subject, D.J.W. spared his audience none of the intricate stages in developing a vaccine: of blowing glass to make pipettes, of the complexities of chemical analysis, of collecting blood serum and making bacterial emulsions, of preparing and staining slides so that bacteria could be counted, of the preparation of a vaccine, and of the negative and positive phases which could occur in the vaccination process itself. His audience must have been somewhat relieved when he moved from the minutiae of laboratory techniques to discussing case studies so as to demonstrate the effectiveness of the inoculation treatment, gory details and all.

The entire subject was radically new to most of his audience. Yet, as one friend commented, he ended his address in a characteristically modest manner, saying:

As a worker in only one narrow department of medicine, I must necessarily have been speaking to many or all of you on matters concerning which your information is more extended and accurate than my own. You must therefore be lenient of my errors and inaccuracies, and let me offer in extenuation my desire to see this valuable means of treatment no longer entirely neglected in the Cape Colony, and I hope by awakening your interest in it, you will proceed to emulate the excellent results achieved elsewhere and by others.

According to Dr. Barnard Fuller, the presentation created a sensation among his colleagues, and was greatly valued as a scientific contribution to a comparatively new and important subject. (8) The complete text of the lecture was published in the *SAMR* for further study.

With a steady stream of articles being published in medical journals together with the presentation of papers, D.J.W. became widely known among the medical fraternity at the Cape. When he stood for the old Cape Colonial Medical Council he had a record vote. From 1906 up to the time of his death he served firstly on this Council, and then, from 1928 on, as a member of the newly formed South African Medical Council (SAMC). In evaluating his contributions over the years, Du Toit felt that although he did not possess great eloquence as a speaker, he spoke out of conviction and 'was always able to state his findings and conclusions clearly and with confidence, without any disagreeable self-assertion, so that he was always a very pleasant colleague to consult with'. (9)

His involvement with these various bodies was no sinecure as he was fully committed to seeing fair play in the medical world. One of his many services to the profession was his sustained fight on behalf of the District Surgeons in the early 1900s. No sooner had he been elected to the Colonial Medical Council than he began to investigate their grievances. At his insistence, the Colonial Secretary agreed to remove one of their biggest complaints, the non-payment for extra work done in

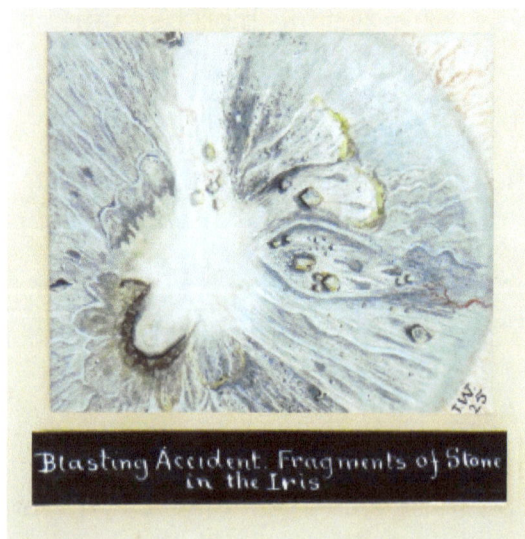

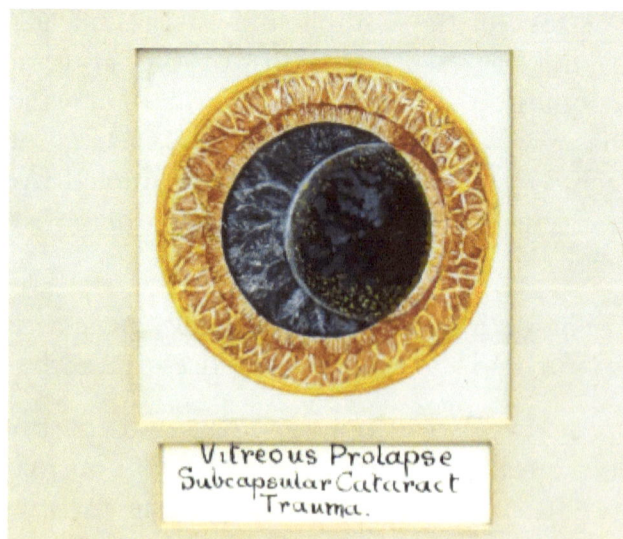

Two signed watercolour paintings, 1925. Left: 'Blasting accident. Fragments of stone in the Iris'. Right: 'Vitreous Prolapse Subcapsular Cataract Trauma' (26)

connection with martial law and military prisoners during the Anglo-Boer War. Assured of this undertaking D.J.W. decided to let the matter rest. But then the plot thickens. In an attempt to muster popular votes in an upcoming election to the Medical Council, and to unseat D.J.W. as his rival, a Dr. J. Hewatt began stirring up trouble amongst the District Surgeons. While trying to rally them into a more confrontational mode, Hewatt represented D.J.W. as being hostile to their ongoing movement to improve their official status.

Meanwhile, in recognition of his active support of the District Surgeons, they had wanted to elect him as Vice-President of their newly formed Association. This information was suppressed by his adversaries. At any rate, he declined the invitation as he was not one of them. In a strongly worded letter to the *SAMR* in June 1903, he protested against the unfair manner in which he had been reported in connection with the whole wretched affair. In a blow-by-blow account he did not hesitate to expose Hewatt's electioneering ploys, which were devious in the extreme. When it came to an attack on his integrity he was no pushover. The editor of the journal published an apology. (10)

True to his philosophy of embracing the medical profession as a whole, D.J.W. moved on from District Surgeons to supporting dentists. At a combined meeting of the Cape branch of the B.M.A. and the Dental Society of the Cape Province in June 1914, he gave a substantial paper on 'Oral and Intestinal Sepsis in Relation to the Diseases of Ophthalmic Patients'. He was delighted that these disparate specialities had come together to share their knowledge. The paper and the discussion were published in both the *Dental Supplement* and the *SAMR*. (11)

In D.J.W.'s own practice he could cite innumerable cases where oral sepsis was either known or suspected to be the cause of various eye diseases. In younger children he had found that tooth decay resulting from defective nutrition was a common cause of corneal ulcers, as was the children's stunted growth. Removal of teeth and cleansing the mouth generally resulted in a good recovery. The parents of a seven-year old boy had needed some persuading to allow his offending teeth to be removed. This had led to a dramatic recovery of eyesight as well as appetite. D.J.W. commented that the old saying 'Better an empty house than a bad tenant', was true even in medicine.

With older patients he identified the regular occurrence of a three-way correlation between oral sepsis in the gums and teeth (associated with toxaemia from some part of the digestive system); rheumatism, pyorrhoea, gout and fibrositis; and a number of different eye diseases. The most common eye ailment was irido-cyclitis, but central choroiditis, ocular paralysis, and senile cataracts could all be related to bad oral sepsis. Some cases of conjunctivitis with ulcers were also suspect.

In those past mid-life and older, the cases tended to be more severe, resulting in secondary cataracts, detachment of the retina, or shrinking of the eye. Any improvement by removing the teeth tended to be limited to general health. Even successful cataract operations in the elderly had been negated by septic teeth. D.J.W. kept meticulous records of his cases but he felt that statistical evidence was needed to ratify his findings.

Chapter 16
A Granddaughter's Treasure Hunt

On his death my grandfather bequeathed his entire collection to the Ophthalmology Department at the UCT Medical School. For many years much of this material was still used as a teaching aid with students. Then it was stored away. Since I started work on this biography, it has been a treasure hunt to try and locate what is left of this precious legacy, more than seventy-five years later. These historic artefacts well illustrate how D.J.W. made best use of what knowledge and equipment were available to him at the time, and of his scientific methods. For me, tangible contact with what was central to my grandfather's life and work has been an emotional experience and a joyful discovery.

In 2009, the treasure hunt started with Professor 'Kay' de Villiers. Thanks to him, some precious finds were located in the Cape Medical Museum. (1) Established in 1982, the museum eventually found a permanent home in the former residence of the Medical Superintendent of the now defunct City Hospital for Infectious Diseases. (2) The Victorian house, painted a rather alarming pink, cannot be missed opposite the UCT Graduate School of Business. When Professor de Villiers started gathering together display material, some of it came from small private collections while the rest was given by 'interested and kindly disposed doctors'. (3)

The wide range of memorabilia records the history of medicine at the Cape, from the indigenous healing herbs of the early hunter-gatherers, to bones still used by Xhosa *sangomas*, through the pioneering days of modern medicine until we reach the present day. Included in the display are original items from D.J.W.'s historic collection that had long been forgotten at Groote Schuur, gathering dust.

In the museum, reconstructions of sets dating from the Victorian days provide a graphic portrayal of the primitive conditions under which my grandfather worked. They also give some idea of his achievements when one considers the limited facilities of the time. A doctor's consulting room is complete with the traditional black bag and a wooden box containing a mobile dispensary, once used by a Riversdale doctor doing his rounds on horseback. A Victorian dental surgery has a cast-iron chair, a manual foot pump, treadle drill and basic dental instruments. There is also an old operating theatre with chloroform and stainless steel hacksaws used during amputations, together with a typical hospital ward. The dispensary, dating from the early 20th century, is lined with shelves of colourful bottled potions, which I can remember from my childhood. Horrors! (4)

My grandfather's ophthalmological instruments are displayed in a glass case. In a newspaper interview, the first curator, Mrs. Anista Keyser, said that it was a miracle that they had survived for so long.(5) The delicate ivory-handled eye operation instruments, still in their original case, show careful craftsmanship. As ivory goes yellow under hot water, it is a wonder that they have kept their colour, let alone the fact that they were made sterile for operations. The set is said to include eight lens needles and four cataract knives. They would date from the 1880s as D.J.W. would have brought them with him from England. Lachrymal probes are dated around 1930. These instruments would now be valued as antique collectables.

On another shelf is a box of 'Holmgren's Colour Perception Test'. This contains skeins of wool in all colours of the rainbow, which D.J.W. used to test colour blindness. (6) A mismatch, such as choosing blue or violet in the Pink Test would indicate red-blind colour-blindness, while the choice of green or grey would indicate green-blind. (7)

More of my grandfather's bequest is stashed away in cupboards. Here are seven long wooden frames with their sealed glass jars. As at Groote Schuur, they contain pathology specimens of eyes that have been fixed, cross-sectioned, and stained for gross and microscopic examination, all precisely labelled in his spidery black handwriting. There are also glass phials containing various objects, such as chips from a hammer, large iron fragments, and pieces of brass and steel, which he had extracted from eyes. The contents of all these containers are recorded in two books, as well as notes on cards. In addition, is a Scotometer chart, patients' record charts from 1924 to 1933, letters from English doctors concerning their treatment of colonial patients, and an original typescript of D.J.W.'s paper on 'A Case of Supra-sellar Meningioma'. (8) Treasure indeed.

The only book in the Wood collection is a classic – *The Anatomy of the Eye and Orbit: including the Central Connections, Development, and Comparative Anatomy of the Visual Apparatus* by Eugene Wolff. This is a first edition published by H.K. Lewis and Co. in London, in 1933, with 173 illustrations. After being revised by a succession of authors, in 1997 it was in its 8th edition and was still regarded as the internationally accepted definitive textbook in this field. (9)

My treasure hunt resurfaced after a gap of four years, and a move nearer to Cape Town. I had the amazing experience of attending the 43rd National Congress of OSSA in the Mother City, in March 2013, to listen to the D.J. Wood Memorial lecture given by Dr. Harold Konig. As the first member of the Wood family to attend an OSSA Congress, I was made to feel very welcome and special. Sitting on the podium with Dr. Deon Doubell, OSSA President, I survived being introduced as Dr. Wood's grandmother (much hilarity), and even the remark that I seemed to be 'a character' like my grandmother (not so sure about that). It was such a privilege to be welcomed into the OSSA family and to meet some of their illustrious members. Professor Andries Stulting, as editor of the opthalmological journal, inspired me to drop the historical writing I was doing and get going with this book. For this I am very grateful as it has been an incredibly moving experience.

After the congress I renewed my search for any remaining tangible links with my grandfather. I was greatly blessed because at every turn I met just the right person at just the right moment, each one going out of his way to help me in my pilgrimage. The first step in this journey was seeing some of my grandfather's watercolour paintings, framed together with those of Tinus de Jongh's in the Ophthalmology Department at Groote Schuur Hospital. A source of wonder and delight.

Then in May 2013, Professor Colin Cook and Professor Tony Murray made a series of amazing discoveries in the Ophthalmology Department, like pulling rabbits out of a hat. First came nine more wooden trays with pathological specimens in glass jars, similar to those in the Cape Medical Museum. These are now on display in

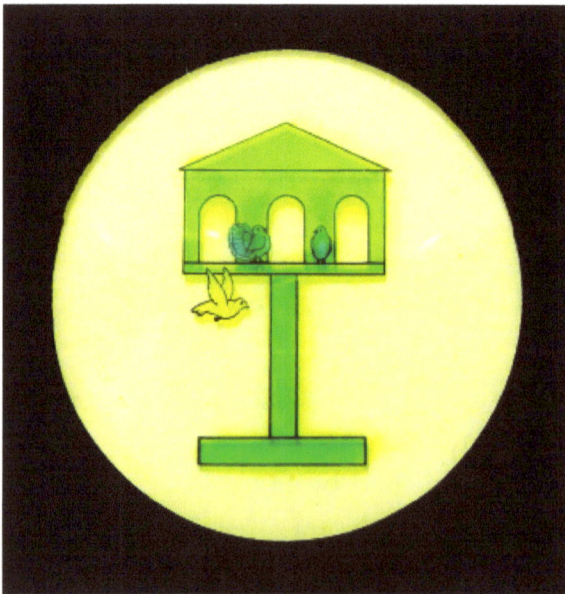

Photographic glass Plate of Dovecote and 3 birds (27)

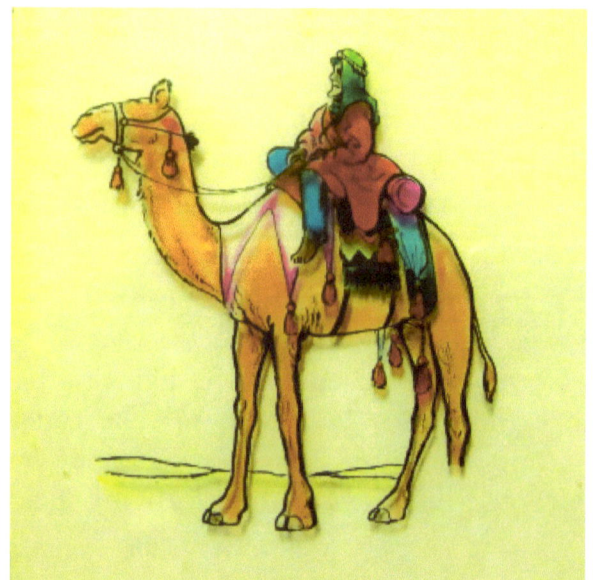

Photographic glass plate of a Camel (28)

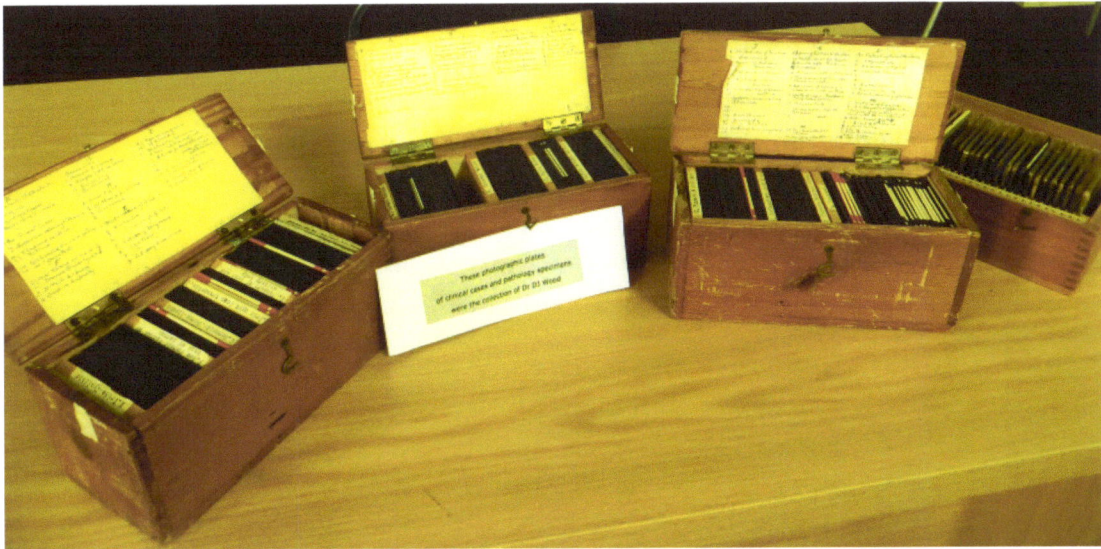

Four boxes of D.J.W.'s Photographic Glass Plates (29)

a glass case in the small ophthalmology museum in the Outpatient Department at Groote Schuur. Then came four wooden boxes containing photographic glass plates, which were miraculously unearthed in the Department's storeroom. The plates, each about ten cm square, record clinical cases and pathology specimens. Dating from the 1920s and 30s, they were projected by a magic lantern.

The contents of each box are listed on the inside of their lids. Some of the slides have labels stuck along their edges, too, grouping them under different headings such as normal and abnormal retina, optic nerve, cornea and iris. Then come examples of diseased eyes - tumours and sections, external viscera, inflammatory conditions, irido-cyclitis, iris cysts, dermoids, tumours of iris ciliary body, new formal tissue on back of cornea, etc. There are also a few photographs of faces with different eye disfigurements, which were used to illustrate articles in the *BJO*.

The longest box holds the biggest surprise of all. Neatly slotted away are a series of pictures on glass plates, imported from England, which D.J.W. used with children. These include a range of coloured imagery – camels, horses, a mouse, two cats, frogs, spiders, spider webs, a dovecot with birds, a pig, a cock, and chickens. Then there are familiar shapes such as a house, little men, a clock, a swing and a couple of flags with contrasting emblems. Lastly, are paintings of shapes such as squares, circles, stripes and spots in different sizes and colours. As a child I have a distant memory of Dr. Townsend trying these out on me, sliding them through some sort of 'scope'. But my lazy eye was a lost cause. I became screwed up with anxiety and nauseous with the desperate effort to see.

As if this was not enough, Professor Murray then uncovered an even more exciting find – a dusty cardboard box with ten of my grandfather's watercolour paintings of diseased eyes, some signed D.J.W. in the corner. How these had eluded earlier searches is a mystery. My daughter-in-law, Julie, has been keeping a photographic record of our treasure hunt so this entailed a fourth visit to Groote Schuur. Professor Cook laid the paintings out in his office for us to marvel at. Some we recognised. Now rather faded, D.J.W. had used them to illustrate papers published in the *BJO*. The paintings have been reframed and hang in the Ophthalmology library.

Together with the paintings was one last memento, which is already hanging in the museum. This is a board with ten glass phials attached to the top. These contain objects, which D.J.W. extracted from eyes, all encased in cotton wool. Stuck below are two typed sheets, brown with age, identifying each item and the method used in extracting it from the damaged eye:

♦ Particle of metal from exploded cartridge embedded in deep layer of cornea: removed with needle.

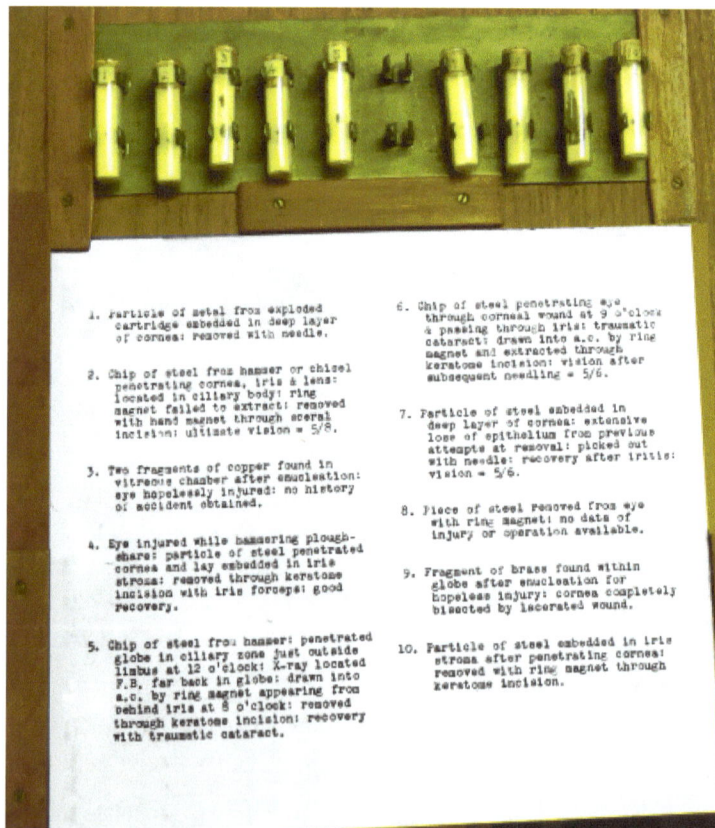

Phials with specimens removed from eyes
mounted on a wooden board with
explanatory notes (30)

- ·Eye injured while hammering ploughshare: particles of steel penetrated cornea and lay embedded in iris: removed through keratome incision with iris forceps: good recovery.

- Chip of steel from hammer or chisel penetrating cornea, iris and lens: located in ciliary body: ring magnet failed to extract: removed with hand magnet through sceral incision: ultimate vision – 5/8

- Two fragments of copper found in vitreous chamber after enucleation: eye hopelessly injured: no history of accident obtained.

- Fragment of brass found within globe after enucleation for hopeless injury: cornea completely bisected by lacerated wound.

On my many visits to the hospital to marvel at these new discoveries, one person who touched my life was the security guard at the boom. Coming from the Breede River Valley himself, he was thrilled to see my CCD car number plate – Robertson to the uninitiated. Besides his kindness in finding me a parking place, when I left he came out of his lodge to give me the Lord's blessing. Sadly, I never asked him his name.

Another recently acquired artefact, quite different from the rest, is a photograph of D.J.W. in one of his beloved Talbots after winning the Siddeley Cup trial in 1912. This is a wonderful memento of his passion for motoring, a century after the event. The faithful September is by his side, our only picture of him. An unidentified couple, probably family members, are seated in the back. This was in accordance with the trial's rules that all the seats had to be occupied. Derek Stuart-Findlay, an authority on classic cars, was the detective in this case. After researching old motoring magazines in the UCT library, my grandfather's photo takes pride of place in his article on the Siddeley Cup, published in *The Crankhandle Chronicle* in June 2013. A second photo shows the line up of cars for the trial with their drivers. The latter included A. Hennessy and J.W. Jagger, family friends and motoring rivals. (10)

For myself, the search to find mementos of D.J.W.'s legacy has been a great adventure. This revered grandparent, about whom I knew almost nothing at the start, has become a living reality and an actual presence in my life. To those who have accompanied me on this journey into the past I express my deepest gratitude. My hope is that part of this unique collection may be put on display at an OSSA congress, or else recorded on the Internet, so that all may share in the many different facets of my grandfather's genius.

✧

PART 5: 'A MASTER OF HIS SUBJECT'

Chapter 17
Founding an Ophthalmological Society

With his reputation as an eye doctor and surgeon standing high, both in South Africa and abroad, D.J.W. was asked to serve on numerous professional committees, was an active member of many Medical Congresses, and was elected president of the ophthalmology sections on several occasions. In 1930, he was also founding father and one of the most active members of the Ophthalmological Society of South Africa (OSSA). This was the first separate society to be formed by any group of medical specialists in South Africa.

In a letter to the *JMASA* in December 1930, headed 'An Ophthalmological Society', D.J.W. reported on the initial attempt of a small group of colleagues to establish such a Society at a meeting of the Medical Association of South Africa in Durban in 1930. (1) Up to that time there had been no way of bringing ophthalmic surgeons together at medical congresses save in 'the spasmodic and sporadic special sections'. The problem was that in the sectional meetings too many specialities with quite different interests were lumped together, with only a small following in each. The result was that the standard of their work was much below that in the medical and surgical sections, something that would have irked D.J.W. immensely. Another difficulty was that officers of sections were chosen locally for each congress, resulting in a varying degree of competence and expertise in any particular subject.

Under such circumstances, there was no possibility of there being any continuity in the aim or practice of those doing ophthalmic work, nor was there any permanent means of establishing a bond between them. D.J.W. found these different issues frustrating and argued convincingly for the importance of having an organization, which was not only concerned with matters primarily of interest to ophthalmic surgeons, but was also indirectly valuable to the public.

Establishing the Society was easier said than done. At the next congress in Durban, because this item was not on the business agenda of the proceedings, discussions had to be sandwiched in at odd times of the day and night. The congress's business meeting was then held before the ophthalmologists were ready to present any kind of report. All the interest group could do was form an interim committee of five. They elected D.J.W. as President, with Dr. A. Verwey in Durban as secretary-treasurer. (2)

Subsequently, D.J.W. drew up a set of draft rules and submitted them to the Medical Council. These were published together with an accompanying letter in the *JMASA*, allowing time for them to be thoroughly digested before being revised at their first meeting. Copies of the draft rules were also sent with application forms to all known ophthalmologists in South Africa. The committee's fervent wish was that they might begin their corporate life with a full quota of members. Mass support was vital to ensure 'a strong and energetic Society'. D.J.W. hoped that many others would join, who, although they did not practise ophthalmology, were still interested in the subject. This would include neurologists, physicians, and others.

He ended his report by begging all ophthalmologists who had not yet joined to send in their application forms as soon as possible. He also made a heartfelt appeal to those who had the management of the forthcoming scientific meeting to waive questions concerning the birth and parentage of the Society, and to assist in sorting out any technical irregularities. A month later he was glad to say that about half of those on their list had already applied. Some had paid a subscription, too, which was used to cover small accounts; but a regular subscription fee would have to be decided on by members at their first meeting.

In a leading article in the same issue of *JMASA*, the editor, Dr C. Louis Leipoldt, came out strongly in support of the ophthalmologists' new venture. As a specialist himself, he understood their need to discuss and consider matters of interest to their own field of medicine. (3) In emphasizing how detrimental professional stagnation in any branch of the medical sciences could be, he reminded his readers of the 3 Cs put forward by Dr. Julius Cohnheim, a German pathologist (1839-1884), many years previously:

These three – consultation, co-operation, criticism – are all-important to the advance of our art and science...Of these three criticism, such as one best obtains in a society where members are so intimately known to each other that the value of their individual opinions can be correctly assessed, is perhaps the most important.

Anticipating any possible resistance to the formation of a highly specialized group, the editor emphasized that the ophthalmologists' meetings would be open to any one interested in their deliberations. Moreover, such a society would be of benefit in broadening their general professional culture as much in the Union as it had been elsewhere. The formation of larger entities, such as the District Surgeons and the Railway Medical Officers Groups, showed how valuable and useful they could be to them all. In addition, the pathologists and the medical officers of health already had sectional groups within the Medical Association. The particular appeal to their members would be the same as with the newly formed Ophthalmological Society.

Like them the Society would encourage criticism, independent and original work, and frank, knowledgeable discussion.

Fortunately, the ophthalmologists were able to negotiate any hurdles and D.J.W. was inducted as President at OSSA's first meeting in September 1931. This was held in conjunction with the S.A.M.C. congress in Pretoria. In his inaugural address he reminded his audience that it was just over fifty years since their parent body in the United Kingdom had come into being, and he expounded on the progress of ophthalmology since then. He trusted that they would follow the dictum of Sir William Bowman, the first President of OSSA in Britain, that their new Society: 'would admit no rivalries within itself, no contentions for rank or credit except those which may establish, under the stamp of time, how much each man may have contributed to develop and advance the whole'.

Bowman had also stressed the importance of active co-operation with colleagues whose interests lay in other medical disciplines. He argued that such associations would 'guard their Society against narrow views and against aims and purposes not worthy of them'. (4) One of the most remarkable aspects of D.J.W.'s medical career was the way in which he embodied this belief to the full. He was generous to a fault in lauding the pioneering work of specialists in other fields, and respectful of conflicting opinions even when they clashed with his own views.

In his presidential address he also expressed the hope that they would elect honorary members whose work was akin to theirs even though they were not medical men. At that time women had yet to make their presence felt. D.J.W. looked forward to the possibility of having lectures 'from men like Gullstrand on optics, Cushing on the relations of the brain and eye, or Del Rio Hortega on modern methods of investigating the structure of the retina'. He was concerned that if they only met once a year to discuss their problems and difficulties they would fall short of their ideal. Two possibilities that still needed to be discussed were the production of an ophthalmological supplement in their medical journal, and the formation of a reference library of books and periodicals that might be covered by a small subscription.

The best news was that out of forty-three ophthalmic surgeons, or those who were partly such, they already had no less than forty members. This was ample proof that such a Society was required, and provided a vote of confidence in their Council for proceeding along the right lines.

Before ending, D.J.W. presented OSSA with a Chairman's gavel and two unique relics. These had an interesting history. During his time as house surgeon at Moorfields, he had found two broken boxes discarded in the cellar. These had held instruments for outpatient work. On one was the name of Sir William Bowman

(1816-1892), foremost as a physiologist of his time and the doyen of British ophthalmology. His work was commemorated each year in the Bowman lecture of OSSA's parent body. On the other box was the name of John Whitakker Hulke (1839-1895), a general surgeon who had specialised in ophthalmic surgery at Moorfields. Hulke, a man of many talents, had also been president of both the British Zoological Society and the Geological Society. (5) D.J.W. had rescued the boxes and had set them on either side of a gavel that was a replica of that presented to the British Ophthalmological Society at its jubilee meeting.

In concluding his presidential address, he said that he trusted that this first birthday of the Society was only the beginning of a long and prosperous career, not only for their mutual benefit, but for that of all mankind. He would be delighted to know that OSSA still honoured these values and had grown from strength to strength.

As the Society developed, business matters were seen to take up an inordinate amount of time at their meetings. Consequently, in 1936 an attempt was made to inaugurate a Clinical Club, focusing on clinical ophthalmology alone. This faded after two years, possibly because D.J.W. was no longer there to keep it going. However, in 1952, ophthalmology was the first medical speciality to publish its own *Transactions*. The Society's meetings were held in conjunction with the annual Congress of the Medical Association and although OSSA had originally intended to remain independent, it eventually became absorbed as a sub-section of the Association. (6)

When D.J.W. formally handed in his resignation as a member of the S.A.M.C. on the day before his death, his colleagues refused to accept it insisting on giving him a year's sick leave. This was a mark of their appreciation for his dedicated commitment to the Council over so many years. At the same time they had greatly valued the clarity and incisiveness of his insight into a wide range of medical matters. (7)

A self-effacing man, my grandfather would have been amazed that OSSA still honours his memory with the giving of the prestigious D.J. Wood Memorial Lecture at their annual Congress. These lectures were begun in 1976 and continue to this day. (8) During his lifetime, D.J.W.'s dedication to extending ophthalmic knowledge and expertise knew no bounds, although he was wont to play down his role as a leader in the field. His family were almost the last to appreciate the esteem in which he was held worldwide, and that was after his death.

Chapter 18
Research and Writing in South Africa

D.J.W. continued with his research right up to the end of his life. With a steady stream of articles being published in medical journals, in South Africa, Britain, North America and the Continent, his clinical work was well known to specialists around the world. As his granddaughter, what interests me most is the person behind the pen. The questions I will be asking, especially in the early years, are about what excited him in ophthalmic breakthroughs? What inspired his never-ending curiosity and sense of adventure? How did he respond to new insights in every field of medicine? How did he overcome his innate humility to pass these new discoveries on so that they could be of benefit to all?

As his research progressed, and his papers became more technical, I find myself in foreign territory. Even so, it has been fascinating to try and fathom the exploratory nature of his work in opening up new frontiers in uncharted fields. Despite my limitations I cannot ignore the versatility of his vision and how he expressed it through his research, because it was so central to his life. Behind the complex observations of a scientific pioneer like D.J.W. was a man of infinite kindness, compassion and love for all who sought his help, no matter their colour or personal circumstances. In trying to reach a wider audience his facility with the written word and his ability to support his findings through a variety of illustrations, resonated far and wide. This chapter is devoted to a brief overview of papers published in South Africa, they being listed for research purposes in Appendix 2.

Shortly after arriving in South Africa, D.J.W. began a series of 'Ophthalmological Notes'. These were published in the *South African Medical Journal (SAMJ)*, founded in 1884. Initially, his focus was on original new work being done in other parts of the world. As the first practising eye specialist in South Africa, his main concern was to keep medical practioners in the country abreast of significant developments, and to suggest how best this information could be utilized. Always modest, he was diffident, if not apologetic, in offering advice. Yet his only wish was to be of service to humanity. This is the common thread running through all his writing.

The first of his 'Notes' was on 'The Use of Eserine in Corneal Disease'. (1) Originally, eserine had proved effective in treating corneal infections but had since fallen out of favour. Drawing on the recent work of Marcus Gunn, his former mentor at Moorfields, it was now said to be superior to atropine in various forms of corneal ulceration, and to have nutritional value in healing the cornea. D.J.W. recommended that a small dosage of drops or ointment should be part of routine treatment in preventing ulceration, as in acute conjunctival inflammations.

The following month he was excited about new physiological research at Moorfields, this time on glands secreting the intra-ocular fluids in the eye. (2) By using microscopic sections to investigate the structure of the iris, and the ciliary body lying just behind it, a former colleague had discovered the 'long-sought-for source' of these fluids in an 'immense number of tubular glands in the ciliary body'. (3) Pathologically, this meant reformulating the diagnoses of some of the most intractable forms of eye disease and offered totally new ways of treating them.

In May 1894, his 'Notes' were again geared to practical issues in eye care. (4) Firstly, it was the use of fluorescein as a stain in examining cases where there was some irregularity of the corneal surface. Not well known in South Africa, one drop of a weak solution was enough to expose non-epithelial elements in the cornea. Abrasions, ulcerated surfaces, etc. could then be instantly and accurately mapped allowing for the correct treatment of the diseased area. In the second part, he reported on American research, which claimed that most epileptics were the subject of refractive errors. Correcting these were said to cure or ameliorate much suffering. He was highly critical of the fashionable treatment, especially in America, with 'spectacles, prisms, or worse still, tenotomies (transection of a tendon or tendon release), so degrading ophthalmic surgery.

In the June issue he dealt with 'Blinding of the Retina from Direct Sunlight'. British research confirmed his experience that 'after images' were common after incautiously looking at the sun: but that real blinding occurred during solar eclipses. The level of permanent damage depended on how long the eyes were subjected to harmful effects in watching the event. Recovery of any vision could take from one to six months. The only treatment was to rest the eyes completely and to protect them from light. Eye damage from exposure to strong sunlight was naturally more prevalent in the southern hemisphere, and his success in treating these cases added much to his reputation. In the same article he discussed recent findings on retinal detachment. These overturned previous beliefs and offered hope for a measure of recovery in what was seen as an incurable disease. (5)

In 1928 he returned to retinal detachment, it being one of an eye surgeon's most difficult problems. (6) Since 1912, he had collected case studies of eighty-seven patients in his private practice, hospital records being too deficient in detail. He also excluded those due to penetrating wounds and tumours. In general, his prognosis and treatment were based on two main causes. Up to now emphasis had been laid on the first, the retina 'being pulled off its attachment by a *vis a fronte*', resulting in a pretty hopeless condition. However, experience had shown that effusion behind the retina, pushing it off, was a more common condition and offered good hope of a 'cure'.

However, good vision depended on many factors. By then he had achieved fourteen 'cures', and in eighteen other cases detachment had remained stationery for up to ten years. For him, getting a case early was half the battle, as any eye surgeon would agree. Besides this, a clear vitreous and a good tension were the most favourable points. Rest came first as a curative agent. This had to be complete and prolonged, with both eyes covered and no movement allowed, a challenge to most patients. Operations to withdraw subretinal fluid were still in the experimental stage, but he thought that they could be combined with injecting normal saline, or a bubble of sterile air into the vitreous.

In his July 1894 'Notes', D.J.W. dealt with infective ulceration of the cornea because of its frequency in lost or impaired vision, and because of the many rival modes of treatment. With the majority of cases coming from local injury, his treatment was three-fold - to remove all possible fresh sources of contagion, to improve the tone of the corneal tissues (by applying warmth through frequent bathing with hot water or with dry heat), and to destroy germs in the infected area. Directions were given for each phase in the process. (7) The last of the 'Ophthalmic Notes' appeared in May 1895. These consisted of brief reviews of the work of French and German ophthalmologists regarding diseases of the retina and cornea, and in passing on suggested treatments. (8)

Whilst D.J.W. still wished to keep colleagues informed about recent research overseas,

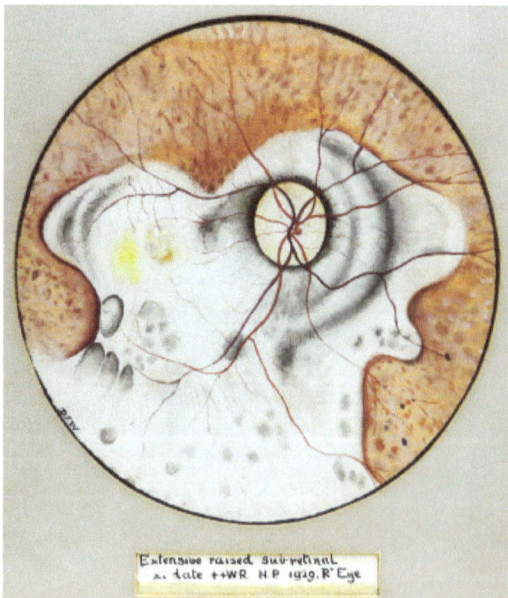

Signed painting by D.J.W.,
'Extensive Raised Subretinal
Exudate++WR H.P. 1929 Rt. Eye'
(31)

by July 1895 he had begun relating this material to his own findings. His South African publications can be divided into two categories. The first are papers read at medical meetings, conferences and symposia, some addressing the medical field in general and others a more specialized audience. The majority of these talks were given in the early to mid part of his career, gathering momentum as his contributions gained increasing respect. They were then reproduced in local medical journals.

The second category involved pioneering research with an ophthalmic audience in mind. He personally submitted these papers to journals for publication. All but one, on the eye complications of leprosy, date from 1928 on. Some articles were accompanied by a photograph of a diseased eye, a sketch to illustrate a problem, or Scotoma chart readings.

The Scotoma diagrams were used to show areas in the visual field of a patient in which vision is absent or diminished, and were dated to demonstrate the progression of the disease and its response to treatment. The artwork was all his own.

The common factor in both categories of writing was that they were based on painstaking observations of specific cases. This involved detailed information on the nature of the disease or damage to the eye, the results of medical examinations to identify related causes, the whys and wherefores of the treatment given, and the outcome, both positive and

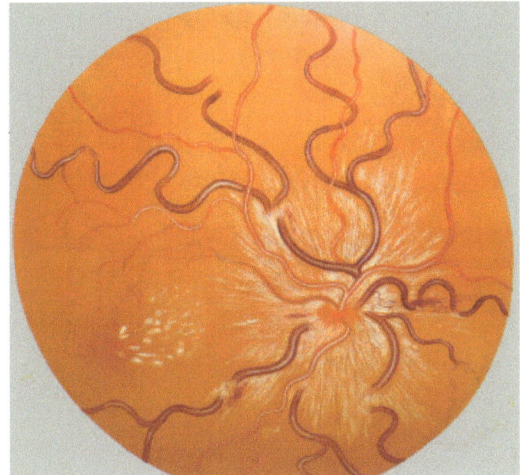

Signed painting by D.J.W. of 'Papilloedema' (32)

negative, over a period of time. The whole process was supported by laboratory research and comparisons with work being done overseas. By keeping his finger on the pulse of developments elsewhere, he was always ready to try new treatments that might prove successful. His papers raised questions, too, about the need for further areas of study and experimentation.

Examples in the first category, published either in the *South African Medical Journal (SAMJ)* or the *South African Medical Record (SAMR)* include a short paper read before the Cape of Good Hope Branch of the BMA in July 1895, where he reported on 'Hereditary Specific Iritis' in a two-year old girl. (9) This was a sad case as the child had all the symptoms of inherited syphilis as indicated by the rapid progression of her diseased eyes. He did not think she would survive long. A year later, he addressed the same group on two cases of eye diseases – 'Ciliary Staphyloma and Opthelmia Neonatorium'. The patients were present providing added interest. (10) His next offering was his inaugural address as President of the Branch in 1906 when he spoke about vaccines. There is then a gap until the combined conference with dentists in 1914.

In 1922, he was asked to introduce a discussion on 'Injuries and Common Diseases of the Eye' at the South African Medical Congress in Johannesburg. (11)) In a major presentation he chose eye conditions of interest to all, and offered much practical advice. He began with the subject of opthalmia neonatorium as it caused so much blindness in babies, the G.P. generally getting the blame. Firstly, the mother needed to be cured of her gonococcal infection before termination of pregnancy. Infection in the baby was avoided by specialised ophthalmic nursing. Midwives must be barred! He then turned to the virulence of gonorrhoeal conjunctivitis in young girls and adults. Constant irrigation of the eyes was needed if sight was to be saved. Most of the paper, however, focused on the various causes of iritis and its treatment This was not only a common problem in general practice, arising from an amazingly wide range of diseases from syphilis, infective jaundice, and septic tonsils to bronchitis, but one which required close collaboration with other specialists.

Three years later, he addressed the 20th S.A. Medical Congress on 'Some Cases of Retinal Disease associated with Streptococcic infection'. (12) Blood tests had shown that the sudden onset of blindness in six young people was of septic origin of low virulence. The infection came from diseased tonsils or pharynx, and was carried by the bloodstream to the retina as an embolus, resulting in permanent loss of some vision. Paintings of the diseased retinae were used as illustrations. Significantly, similar cases had yet to be linked together and reported in the international literature.

That same year, 1925, he presented two papers to the local branch of the BMA. The first, on the Co-ordimeter of Professor Ness, was about a simple apparatus designed by a physiologist in Zurich to give accurate detection and diagnosis of the paralysis of an eye muscle. (13) In the second paper, he explained the importance of optic neuritis, or papillaedema, in diagnosing intracranial tumours. As it was not an inflammatory condition and could not occur without organic disease, it was one of the early signs of a tumour but was easy to miss. (14)

From 1928 on, D.J.W.'s articles in local journals were all research-oriented, based on case studies and laboratory work, which he submitted himself. The one on retinal detachment came first. This was followed by eight more papers before his death in 1937. These were published either in the *Journal of the Medical Association of S.A. (B.M.A.)* or the *S.A. Journal of Medicine/ S.A. Tydskrif vir Geneeskunde.*

A number of these scientific studies were illustrated in various ways. In 1931, his article on glaucoma included two Scotoma Charts showing the dark shapes of the paracentral scotomata. (15) Whilst in a study of Supra-sellar Meningioma in 1936, the Scotoma charts were accompanied by a photograph. (16) Again a photo gives the general appearance of the eye in his paper on the staining of the cornea by blood-pigment, but a sketch is added to show ruptures of the iris. (17)

Other original contributions in the 1930s included a paper on fundus conditions in which he identified seven distinct varieties of white dots. Having seen many such cases, he believed that they were essentially different in prognosis, appearance (brilliance and arrangement), and etiology. (18) Despite failing health, he continued to publish a flurry of research papers. A short one in 1936 provided clinical notes on avulsion of an eye, (19) while a longer one was on trachoma problems. (20)

Trachoma took him back to the founding of Moorfields in 1805 to deal with the diseased eyes of British troops returning from Egypt. D.J.W. noted that Egypt was still the country *par excellence* where trachoma could be studied as the disease was universal among the peasantry and very common even among the higher classes, causing regular epidemics of conjunctivitis. Because it was contagious he argued that immigrants from such countries should be checked on arrival. Those with trachoma should be refused entry or else treated effectively under the Health Department's supervision so as to stamp out the disease in South Africa before it could spread.

But it was his literary scholarship as much as his scientific discoveries, as in his monograph on the blindness of John Milton, that so impressed his colleague and editor of the *SAJM*, Dr. C. Louis Leipoldt.

Chapter 19
Dr. C. F. Louis Leipoldt, Editor and Colleague

Dr. Christian Frederic Louis Leipoldt was twenty-five years my grandfather's junior, and came from a completely different background. Yet the two were not only colleagues on the staff of the New Somerset Hospital and lecturers at the UCT Medical School, but they worked closely together for the S.A. Medical Association and its journal, and became good friends.

Leipoldt was the grandson of a German Rhenish missionary, who founded the mission station at Wuppertal. His father started off as a Rhenish missionary, too, and was assisting his father-in-law in Worcester when Louis was born in December 1880. Four years later his father had joined the Dutch Reformed Church and become the Rev. C.F. Leipoldt. The family then moved to Clanwilliam where Louis was brought up. His mother would not allow her sons to attend school or mix with local children, and so they were taught by their father, a scholarly man with a well-stocked library, and a talented violinist.

Louis received a liberal education, which included French, Greek, and Latin. His home languages were Cape Dutch, German and English. He was also exposed to Eastern religions thanks to his father, who had served as a missionary in Sumatra, a region with strong ancient Buddhist roots side by side with Islam. Louis himself visited Southeast Asia as an adult. No wonder, then, that he later turned to Buddhism.

From an early age Louis took a special interest in botany. He collected specimens of indigenous flora for leading South African botanists like Harry Bolus, as well as imbibing knowledge of healing plants from a traditional African diviner. He also started writing as a youngster. At fourteen he was already contributing articles to newspapers in the Cape. Once he had passed his matriculation and Civil Service examinations in the late 1890s, he became a full-time journalist in Cape Town. In 1902 Bolus lent him the money to go to England to study medicine at Guy's Hospital in London, but he continued with his writing to augment his income.

In 1907 he obtained the M.R.C.S. and the L.R.C.P. and was awarded gold medals for both medicine and surgery. After qualifying he studied the diseases of children, gaining a fellowship of the Royal College of Surgeons. This was followed by various hospital posts, working as a ship's doctor, and as a medical inspector of schools in London. In between he travelled widely on the Continent and Southeast Asia, writing all the time.

In 1914, he passed his F.R.C.S. examination at the second attempt and returned to South Africa. With the outbreak of war he was drafted into the army and became personal doctor to General Louis Botha for a time. But from 1914 until the end of 1922 his administrative post was as Medical Inspector of Schools in the Transvaal. He then went back to writing and became assistant editor of *Die Volkstem*.

Three years later he left journalism to settle in Cape Town and take up work as a children's specialist. Never the less, he continued to write all his life, in English and in Afrikaans. His prodigious output embraced poetry, plays, novels and history, as well as health matters, dietetics, cookery, food and wine. (1) He perfected his gourmet cooking skills under the tutelage of a large Malay woman in the White House Hotel kitchen in Cape Town. She is said to have prodded him with a wooden spoon whenever he made a mistake. (2)

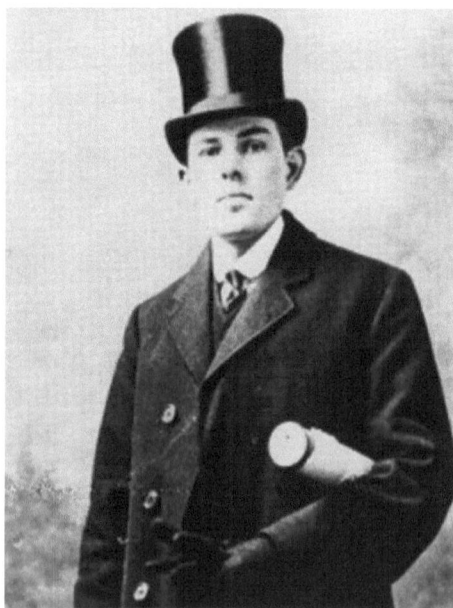

Dr. F.C. Louis Leipoldt (33)

In 1926 he became the first organising secretary of the Medical Association of South Africa and the first editor of their journal, holding both posts until the end of 1944. Before long he added the alternative Afrikaans title of *Suid-Afrikaanse Tydskrif vir Geneeskunde* to the *S.A. Medical Journal*. (3) In 1927 he was appointed a part-time staff member of the UCT Medical School. He was their first lecturer in children's diseases with an honorarium of one hundred pounds per annum. (4) That same year he was given a part-time post at the New Somerset Hospital, where he started to work alongside D.J.W.

Leipoldt was said to be unkempt in appearance, slightly stooped, with unruly bushy hair. He always carried a large Gladstone bag and was an inveterate pipe smoker, favouring Magaliesberg tobacco. His manner was provocative and unpredictable. He was outspoken in his opinions to the point of rudeness and, like my grandmother, did not suffer fools gladly. As the first consultant in children's diseases he had something of an uphill struggle among his medical colleagues. They were of the opinion that 'this was the least necessary of all specialities, every doctor knew about children, or children were the easiest and simplest of patients'. (5) But he persevered and put paediatrics on the map in South Africa.

As editor of the *SAMJ*, Leipoldt wrote a long and affectionate tribute to my grandfather after his death. This is quite unlike any other in that it gives a more rounded view of his personality and honours his gifts in so many different fields. (6) Only someone like Leipoldt, endowed with a free and pioneering vision could, as a eulogist, do justice to the broad sweep of D.J.W.'s humanity, scientific acumen and life's mission.

Leipoldt recalled that he had first come into contact with D.J.W., not as a colleague, but as a young journalist on 'a paper whose opinions must have been anathema to the doctor. Yet I found him courteous and kind, though refreshingly outspoken and very determined in his opinions'. Leipoldt's early journalism in Cape Town had been on the pro-Rhodes newspapers, *De Kolonist* and *Het Dagblad*. After the outbreak of the Second Anglo-Boer War, however, he had become the Dutch correspondent for the pro-Boer *South African News*, very much on the other side of the fence to the Anglophile D.J.W.

After Leipoldt returned to the Cape in 1914, he met up again with D.J.W., and spoke warmly of their renewed acquaintance and close fellowship:

'A very kindly, informative and interested colleague. From that time I think I may boast of his friendship, but my relations with him became more intimate when I started practice in Cape Town in 1926, and took over the editorship of the journal. It was always a pleasure to watch him demonstrate or expound a case. His interest was so manifest, his enthusiasm so genuine, and his knowledge so accurate, that one felt he was a master of his subject. He was very popular with his patients, even those who resented his rather curt way and his political opinions'.

According to Leipoldt, D.J.W. had as wide a reputation among his patients as he had among the colleagues of his own specialty: The latter recognised in him an enquiring and original mind and a forcible critic. The former found in him a most gentle, sympathetic and humane man and friend. Leipoldt remembers how many of D.J.W's patients, who had nothing wrong with their eyes, would still come to him for advice as to whom they should go and see for a particular ailment. As editor of the medical journal, Leipoldt was even more appreciative of D.J.W.'s support as an active contributor of high quality material, and for his masterly grasp of the English language:

He was one of those who could be relied upon to produce a manuscript, whether it was on an original theme, a clinical case, or a comment on someone else's paper. He always expressed himself in fluent, clear and concise English. He hated circumlocution and those incongruities that are the bane of a medical journalist's life, and whose correction worries a medical sub-editor into an early grave. Not for him were the patients 'cases'; nor did they 'run a temperature'; not for him was any 'eye disease' due to something bacteriological or anything else. He was incapable of writing the sort of English with which, unfortunately, medical students are becoming increasingly familiar through the slipshod methods of medical writers. His English style he owed to his passionate fondness for and love of good English, for he was one of those who held Milton and Wordsworth among the ancients, and Trevelyan and Bridges among the moderns, in high esteem.

Robert Bridges was Poet laureate in Britain from 1913 to 1930. Leipoldt was reminded of D.J.W.'s enthusiastic response to Bridges' publication of 'A Testament of Beauty'. In an animated discussion of certain of its aspects, he had been especially appreciative of 'its melodiousness and assonantic rhythm'. Although D.J.W. was not on the regular reviewing staff of the journal, he would send them reviews of anything that interested him. One particularly fine review had been on the standard work on Milton's blindness, an article that was extensively quoted and excerpted from by the American and Continental medical press. The article was reprinted as a monograph with the November 23rd issue of the *SAMJ* in 1935. As to D.J.W.'s contributions to the old *Medical Record* and to the newer *SAMJ*, Leipoldt had nothing but praise. As editor, he appreciated the fact that they were marked by 'a high degree of literary excellence, by originality, and by the thoroughness with which he verified his premises and facts'.

D.J.W. was particularly well known for his keen interest in the histological and pathological side of ophthalmology, and for his skill with microphotography. Leipoldt maintained that his photomicrographs were gems of beauty. The only difference of opinion they had ever had was in Leipoldt's capacity as editor when they had had to discuss the reproduction of 'those beautiful bits of work'. Leipoldt had much regretted having to tell his brilliant colleague that unfortunately the journal's resources were unable to reproduce them with the same faultless accuracy and the same vivid intensity as shown by the originals. D.J.W. had remained unconvinced until the editor had demonstrated how differences of glazing and quality of paper, together with pressure, influenced the reproduction of a zincograph. As he left the office D.J.W. had remarked, in his characteristically dry manner: 'It is high time you got some modern resources in this office'.

With reference to D.J.W.'s services to the Cape of Good Hope (Western) Branch of the British Medical Association, Leipoldt recalled that he gave equally of his best. He had served as President and long-time member of the Council, and regularly attended all the meetings: 'His criticism was always instructive, pertinent and knowledgeable, and his opinion was therefore received with respect'. Leipoldt believed that D.J.W.'s life would stimulate and inspire all those whom he had helped in their career as doctors and who under his leadership had had the opportunity of studying his character and his methods. (7)

Chapter 20
'The Blindness of John Milton'

D.J.W.'s article on the blindness of John Milton is based on a monograph on the subject by a blind American lady, Mrs. Eleanor Gertrude Brown. She had written it as a thesis for a doctorate degree from Columbia University. In his review D.J.W. adds much of his own thinking, especially his diagnosis of the most probable cause of Milton's blindness. (1) Having teased out all available information he came to a reasoned conclusion that upset popular theories, and made people around the world take note of him as a serious literary and medical critic.

D.J.W. began by arguing that Milton's poetry – not to mention his prose - had become neglected because of the considerable demands it made on a classical education. With his scholastic Scottish upbringing, D.J.W. had no problem in translating Milton's letters direct from Latin. 'Even Satan,' he said, 'by far the most impressive figure in "Paradise Lost", has fallen on evil days, though there be still some like the old Scot who boldly said, "for a releegion without a Deevil I would not gie a damn."' As to Homer, few could now read this other great blind poet, 'and the music of his hexameter has never been rendered into a modern tongue'.

For D.J.W. not only did Milton, the greatest English epic poet, still have the power to stir the imagination, and to impress with his unrivalled command of English, but 'for one particular section of mankind, those who cannot see, he remains a joy, an encouragement, and an inspiration'. There is no doubt as to my grandfather's compassion for blind people. The article also gives some idea of the breadth of his knowledge, providing us with a unique insight into his values, beliefs, literary prowess, love of history, and dry sense of humour, as well as his medical expertise.

His review begins with an historical overview of the period in which John Milton lived (1608-1674). It was a time in which the first flower of the Renaissance was beginning to pass, and 'the virile force of the Reformation was spending itself in theological controversies, its purity soiled by prostitution to political aims, and its dream of a universal Protestant Church dead'. The Church of Rome was regaining lost ground, and James I, 'the last of the Scottish Kings and their sorriest specimen', was on the throne. Although the Renaissance had given birth to many men of ability, learning and enterprise, such as Raleigh, Bacon and Shakespeare, science in general had remained rudimentary. Medical science had made minimal progress and was at a very low ebb, with 'much of its pharmacopoeia little better than the ingredients of a witches' cauldron'.

Milton was born in Cheapside, London. His father was a scrivener, as a public notary who wrote out deeds was called in 16th century Scotland. He was said to be a good lawyer, an accomplished gentleman, a musician of parts and a scholar. John had all the advantages of an excellent education and became a master of Latin, the *lingua franca* of Europe, as well as Greek, Hebrew, French and German. He started writing poetry from an early age and rarely left his studies before midnight. His family was Puritan, but not in 'the terrible creed of John Calvin'. Milton later rejected Calvinism completely. Music, an occasional visit to the theatre, and 'various manly sports', such as the use of the broadsword, provided acceptable recreation. Even in his youth, however, Milton knew that he had poor sight and suffered much from headaches. D.J.W, thought this was probably due to the customary diet of meat and pastries, and his sedentary life.

Milton took his B.A. and M.A. degrees at Cambridge. He intended to enter holy orders but could not abide the petty details, ritual and policies, backed by statutory oaths enforced by the Puritan-baiting Archbishop of Canterbury, William Laud (1573-1645). Milton was not a man to stand coercion in matters of conscience, and was, as he says, 'church outed by the prelates'. After leaving college he spent a year in Italy where 'he was welcomed for his scholarship, but disliked by the clergy for his opinions, perhaps resulting from his visit to Galileo, then in prison'. Meanwhile things had gone from bad to worse in England. The King's untrammelled leadership aroused deep feelings of resentment until his death. Despite some reforms, his son's upbringing had foredoomed him to disaster, too.

Amidst these troubled times, Milton, now thirty, married the daughter of a Gay Cavalier house. She could not handle the seriousness, high thinking and hard work of her new life and went home after a month, refusing to return. Milton responded by publishing a treatise on divorce, incurring the condemnation of the clergy. But he was not unkind, and when Oliver Cromwell's reign had spelt ruin to his wife's family he took her back. She remained until her death in 1652, leaving him with three daughters. During the Civil War he took the side of the Puritans, 'his pen being far more potent than would have been his sword'. He was rewarded with a State appointment under the Commonwealth, but, with his sight gradually deteriorating, he eventually had to resign.

The execution of Charles I soured foreign relations and Milton was called in by the Government to write a response to a damaging French pamphlet. He accepted the task as a sacred duty knowing that it would end all hope of saving the remainder of his sight. By 1652 he was not only blind, but had to contend with slander against his opinions. In 1656 he married again, the romance of his life; but his wife died in childbirth fifteen months later. Reconciled to blindness, he now turned his thoughts to an 'inward light'. Yet feeling that his household needed a head, he married once more. This was a colourless relationship, but kindness made his latter days comfortable and he died peacefully in 1674 from an attack of gout.

Besides many prose works, now mostly forgotten, Milton wrote his three great epics, 'Paradise Lost', 'Paradise Regained', and 'Samson Agonistes', all after he became blind. He believed that blindness had helped his imagination. In her thesis, Dr. Brown spoke of three periods in the life of those who become blind – depression, resignation, and, in most, a desire to overcome the handicap. Blind herself, she said that but for the advent of patience in the second stage the blind would go mad. She quotes from Book II in 'Paradise Lost', saying that this is not a lament but a hallelujah:

Hail, holy light, offspring of Heaven first born...

So much the rather thou Celestial light,

Shine inward, and the mind through all her powers

Irradiate, there plant eyes; all mist from thence

Purge and disperse, that I may see and tell

Of things invisible to mortal sight.

D.J.W. comments that 'all of us know how in darkness we may get light on problems which in the distraction of day have evaded solution'. Dr. Brown claimed that people who lost their sight after about seven years of age still saw in their dreams. In a sonnet Milton describes how in a dream his saintly second wife appeared to him. She was veiled, he never having seen her face. She bent over to embrace him but then he woke - 'she fled, and day brought back my night'.

In trying to explain the reason for his blindness, Milton thought that in his youth he had caused excessive strain on his eyes, which were already congenitally defective, by reading well past midnight by the flickering light of candles. He later wondered whether it was his staunch Puritan faith that was the problem: that God was punishing him for his radical political and ecclesiastical views. He readily concurred with many of his influential friends that God had inflicted him with total blindness for his unholy alliance with Oliver Cromwell, a rabid Republican, who had so irreverently flouted the sacrosanct precept of kingship as being of divine origin and ordained by divine fiat. However, both Dr. Brown and D.J.W. are silent as regards Milton's beliefs on divine retribution as the cause of his blindness.

Based on the meagre data available, Dr. Brown set down the prevailing theories on Milton's blindness from a medical point of view. D.J.W. contends that many were either impossible or incredible nonsense, such as 'one weird theory that it was a case of albinism'. He summarily dismisses Milton's own idea that it was due to the excessive use of his eyes in study, saying that it found echo in a belief that was still around. Based on known facts of the poet's symptoms, D.J.W. explains exactly why it could not have been due to cataracts or congenital factors. He also discounts optic atrophy and inherited syphilis, there being no family history of the latter. The two real possibilities were chronic glaucoma and myopia (short-sightedness) leading to retinal detachment.

The only description Milton gave of his trouble was in a letter to a Greek friend written in 1654 in Latin, which D.J.W. translated. After mentioning some digestive problems, Milton said that when he started reading in the morning he immediately felt a pain deep in his eyes. Mild bodily exercise helped, but when he looked at a candle a sort of halo appeared to replace it. Not long after this a dark cloud arose on the left side of the left eye (the one that failed first), which blotted out everything on that side. If he closed his right eye objects in front appeared to be reduced in size.

After considering this evidence, D.J.W. is certain that the symptoms are not characteristic of glaucoma. Others had attached much importance to the presence of halos seen round the candle; but Milton does not use the word *redimire*, to encircle, but *redimere*, to redeem or replace. The main prop of the popular glaucoma theory then falls away and with it the rest of the symptoms that had been twisted to fit the encircling halos. Moreover, one of the pitfalls of early glaucoma was that a person was not aware of his loss of visual field until it became great. This was due to the damage to the optic nerve fibres, which conducted the impressions to the brain. He would never experience a sensation of blackness because this was due either to damage to the rods and cones of the retina (as in early choroiditis), to detachment of the retina (where they are torn through), or where there is an opacity in front of them (as in a haemorrhage).

Milton was a careful observer. He says that when he became blind and went to bed he saw all sorts of coloured appearances - phosphenes or photopsiae. At first they were brilliant and vivid in colour, but as time passed they became degraded and darker. This was common in detachment of the retina but almost unheard of in glaucoma. Other symptoms such as faint luminous sensations provided added evidence, while the pain deep in the eye suggested advancing myopia. In contrast, the glaucoma ache was usually felt at night or after much use of the eyes.

Curiously enough, since beginning the review D.J.W. had had a patient with similar symptoms to Milton, which made diagnosis more credible. However, it was not yet fully understood why even in moderate degrees of myopia there were associated changes in the choroid and secondarily in the retina. The latter was doubtless due to some failure of the blood supply to the rods and cones so that their function was interfered with. Should there be damage in the yellow spot region, which was not actually destructive, there might be oedema. By spacing out the macular cones, this caused the sensation of micropsia — objects seemed smaller than they were to the unaffected eye - as Milton had noticed. There was thus a large body of proof that he suffered from progressive myopia in unhealthy eyes, which eventually led to detachment of the retina, first in one eye and then the other. Every ophthlamic surgeon had seen such cases.

D.J.W. also presented collateral evidence to show that short sight was a familial defect. Milton's father could read without glasses into his eighties, meaning that he had myopia in one or both eyes. D.J.W. had had a similar case with a well-known clergyman in Cape Town. This patient had transmitted myopia in both eyes to all his daughters but was unaware of his own defect until his vision had been tested in his seventies. Milton's mother wore glasses when she was thirty, probably because of short sight. The chances were, therefore, that Milton inherited myopia from both parents. This would account for him becoming worse than either. One of his daughters and a granddaughter had also had weak eyes.

No conclusion could be drawn from his writing that he was not short sighted. He himself had said that his eyes were always weak. Further, the presence of myopia would go far to determine his extraordinary love of reading. Myopia tended to lead to studious habits, not the reverse. Dr. Brown believed that there was much in Milton's writing that was autobiographical, as in Sonnet XIX, on his blindness.

When I consider how my light is spent,

Ere half my days in this dark world and wide,

And that one talent which is death to hide

Lodged with me useless, though my soul more bent

To serve therewith my Maker, and present

My true account, lest He returning chide,

'Doth God exact day-labour, light denied?'

I fondly ask. But patience, to prevent

That murmur, soon replies, 'God doth not need

Either man's work or his own gifts. Who best

Bear his mild yoke, they serve him best. His state

Is kingly, thousands at his bidding speed,

And post o'er land and ocean without rest;

They also serve who only stand and wait.

Milton, however, was not one to stand and wait. He composed his great epics from twenty to fifty lines at a time. One of his daughters then had to write these down immediately, often during the night. He never spared himself, and he expected his family to follow suit. Not so the girls. Their father's demands grew irksome so that finally he sent them about their business to learn 'such occupations as are suitable for women'.

D.J.W. thought that Milton's last epic poem, 'Samson Agonistes', was inspired by his own experience: 'Samson, a giant in strength, Milton a giant in intellect, both struck down in the plenitude of their power. Familiar as was Milton with Semitic history and language, the task was easy, but whether the sympathy, and the insight into the feelings of the blind could have been achieved by one who could see, is at least doubtful.'

In the end Milton was not unhappy, though all he had fought for in religion and good government was swept away in the corruption of the Restoration. He kept friends who were worth keeping, and made new ones from those who could appreciate his intellect and assist him. He died at the age of sixty-six and is buried in the churchyard of St. Giles, Cripplegate. In ending his review, D.J.W. says that: 'We cannot but be amazed at his learning and the persistence with which he pursued it, even when he became dependent on others. His command of English is unrivalled, and his classical lore so great that one may be at a loss to follow his allusions'. D.J.W. also commends Dr. Brown for her book, 'As the work of a blind woman who has conquered her handicap, and come out victorious, praise is a supererogation'.

D.J.W.'s investigation of Milton's blindness was unique in that he was able to use his three-edged perspective of a literary critic, a classics scholar and an ophthalmic surgeon with clinical precision. He resisted the lure of being drawn into any theological or metaphysical rationale, while folklore, which held that the poet's love of reading was responsible for his loss of sight, was dismissed out of hand. After thorough research, other fanciful diagnoses were also kicked out of court. D.J.W.'s professionalism and scientific acumen enabled him to focus on the hardcore evidence without any undue distractions. This made the review the standard text on Milton's blindness, justly earning him international recognition.

Chapter 21
Celebrated Beyond South African Shores

As Louis Leipoldt rightly said, D. J.W. was 'a master of his subject'. His articles, which appeared in South African journals, were often addressed to a wider audience at a meeting or conference, and offered practical advice to medical colleagues. In contrast, his papers published in the *British Journal of Ophthalmology (BJO)* were based on clinical studies and scientific research, and were directed at sharing his findings with others in his field so as to push back the frontiers of ophthalmology.

Here again I will only be giving a brief overview of the scope of this work as it is quite outside my competency. As a biographer, my particular interest is in how my grandfather managed to marry the hidden beauty of medical observations presented through his artwork with the cold precision of his factual documentation. Almost a century ago he was moved by the power of a visual presentation to portray the intricate pathology of diseased eyes so that his colleagues might better understand the mysteries he was trying to uncover and so facilitate a better prognosis.

At that time, professional medical artistry was still in its infancy and those like Tinus de Jongh provided anatomical illustrations as required without any interpretation. In contrast, D.J.W. was a surgeon-artist who pioneered the incorporation of medical art and aesthetics as a visual tool in the practice of ophthalmology. (1) Through his sketches, paintings, diagrams, slides and photography he could be regarded as a latter-day Leonardo in his field. This was clearly appreciated by the *BJO* who spared no expense in reproducing his many different illustrations in conjunction with his articles. Moreover, the manner in which he wielded his surgical knife, his artist's brush and his writer's pen with such uncommon ambidexterity won him international fame.

The *BJO* was founded in 1917 and D.J.W. was their much-respected South African representative right from the start. He remained in post for twenty years until his death. (2) In an Obituary, the editor of the *BJO* wrote:

His loss is a heavy one. Hardly a year passed during the life of this journal in which he did not send us at least one paper for publication. His papers were usually clinical in type and a marked feature of them was the illustrations. He did all his own sectioning and micro-photography, and many of the results were of a very high order of merit.

The editor added that Wood's literary efforts were not confined to clinical ophthalmology as exemplified in his paper on Milton and Milton's blindness. He ended by saying that he would miss very much the many kindly letters he had received during the past thirteen years 'from one whom, though unknown personally, he was proud to consider a friend'. (3)

In another *BJO* obituary there is a reference to D.J.W.'s earlier offerings. Harking back to his time at Moorfields Eye Hospital as eye surgeon from 1889 on, he was said to have been 'peculiarly well-fitted for the post of ophthalmic surgeon in any Gun-Shot Injuries, and on Lightning Injuries of the Eye', and to have been an author of a manual of military ophthalmology. There is no other record to substantiate this statement. (4) However, the obituary goes on to mention his many contributions to the *BJO*, and his output was indeed extraordinary. He had at least nineteen papers published in this esteemed journal, between 1920 and 1936, of which I have copies (See Appendix 3).

In 1920, he started with three short articles. The first was about the removal of injured irises. In one, a carpenter had fallen against wire netting, and in another, a fitter was struck in the eye by a piece of iron. (5) The offending objects were placed in sealed jars and labelled for posterity. The second paper was on a detached retina, a theme he returned to a number of times. (6) The last was about eye complaints caused by malaria picked up by travellers in German East Africa, and by those suffering from the deadly influenza epidemic that had raged across the country in 1918, decimating the population. (7) Indeed, most of the papers he submitted to the *BJO* tended to be unusual cases not normally found in Britain but quite common in the southern hemisphere, so providing radical new insights in previously unexplored avenues of ophthalmic research.

Ocular leprosy was one such, and he called it a great tragedy for those who contracted the disease. (8) By 1925 the advent of the slit-lamp and binocular microscope had enabled him to make a more detailed study of patients who were thought presentable enough to come to his clinic from Robben Island. This gave him sustained evidence into the profound changes taking place during the slow progression of the disease, while experimental treatments seemed to be offering some relief. In the same issue he had a paper on hyatid cysts on the orbit of the eye. (9) Although he had seen many such cases, there were few references in the literature. After surgical intervention and further treatment he was amazed by the extraordinary capacity of the affected eye to recover sight after long periods of blindness.

From 1921 on, D.J.W. made the most of the more sophisticated printing technology available in the British journal. He now regularly included sketches, photographs, watercolour paintings, and sections of pathology specimens recorded on glass photographic plates. His skill with microphotography was a boon in illustrating clinical cases. In 1921, he sent a photograph of a young man's face to show blindness in one eye. (10) The following year he drew sketches for two papers. One is of a young woman's eye in which pus had remained in the cornea for twenty years following measles as a child. (11) The other depicts a cystic body on the iris caused by a parasite. This was accompanied by a microphotograph showing the parasite's head and spider-like suckers. (12) But in 1925 he really got going when he provided watercolour paintings of two uncommon cases of non-traumatic cysts of the interior chamber of the eyes of two young girls. One painting was given a whole page to itself and the other, a smaller detail. (13)

An even longer paper in 1927, on a case of sympathetic ophthalmitis, was illustrated with six microphotographs recorded on glass plates. The magnified sections of the optic nerve, various cells and pigments in the iris, and a lymphatic node, must have excited much interest in D.J.W.'s pioneering use of this new technology. (14) He returned to the same subject three years later with two more cases because he felt they made an interesting trio. This time he was given three pages to present twelve incredibly detailed sections of gross disease in the choroid and iris of 'the exciting eye', as well as the infection in 'the sympathising eye', showing how the two cases differed. Each figure was accompanied by an explanatory note indicating the degree of magnification used and points of interest in the section. (15)

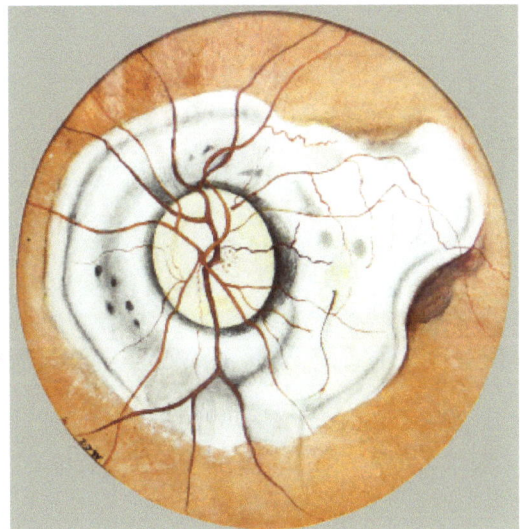

Signed painting by D.J.W., 'Raised sub retinal exudates H.P. Left Eye' (34)

A range of papers followed including the effects of calcium deficiency on eyes, (16) some peculiarities in a patient's iris, (17) glaucoma following thrombosis of the retinal vein (18), a case on traumatic irido-cyclitis, (19) another case on congenital cataract showing unusual features, (20) and observations on the human retina. (21) Almost all the papers were illustrated with sections taken from his glass photographic plates showing the most amazing details. It was exciting for us to see the original plates from which many of these illustrations were taken, the quality of these historic artefacts seemingly intact. Neatly filed and labelled in their boxes, they are now secure in the Groote Schuur Ophthalmological museum.

As D.J.W.'s papers got longer and longer, the reports of each clinical case became ever more detailed. In his presentation he would discuss what the sections were intended to show, what stains were used to highlight different elements and why, what conclusions could be drawn from the evidence, what treatment had been provided, and the results. In the article on the iris, a slit-lamp drawing was also included, while the one on cataracts had paintings of both eyes. These illustrations were all allotted full pages in the journal.

Clearly the *BJO* set great store by the quality of D.J.W.'s graphic artwork and photographic genius. In addition to the meticulous nature of his scientific discoveries, his various illustrations were given an increasingly generous amount of space. He in turn must have been delighted with the quality of the reproductions, adding much to the definitive nature of his observations.

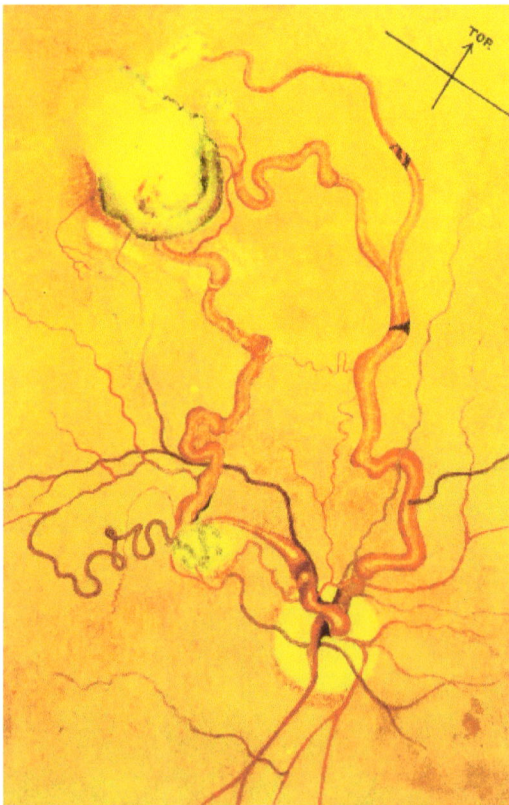

Signed painting by D.J.W., 'Retinal Amacroma (aneurism) (35)

His last article in September 1936 was on inflammatory diseases of the eye caused by gout. (22) Because gout was no longer as common as in the past, he feared that it would be overlooked as a cause or a complication in the production of certain eye diseases. In the last fifteen years he had dealt with four cases with comparable symptoms. As there had been no manifest evidence of gout at the start, more modern aetiologies had been sought, and paid for, without success.

First came a lady who had lived in India. With a wry sense of humour, he noted that 'her husband's position had made hospitality and good living part of his duties, and subsequently she at least had not fallen behind her former habits'. She suffered acute attacks of pain in one eye with red, swollen eyelids, and a prominent eyeball. After seeing three more cases, and with supportive medical tests, D.J.W. was sure that the inflammatory eye disease was caused by gout. The difficulty was in convincing the patient of the problem 'or else he would not take kindly to restrictions of diet, stoppage of alcohol and the discomforts of medication', all of which had proved successful in treatment. This time an account of the abnormalities in the diseased eyes was accompanied by seven pages of enlarged microphotographs of pathogenic sections.

In 1937, D.J.W.'s pioneering work over forty years was recognised by being the first South African ophthalmologist to be invited to deliver the Doyne Memorial Lecture at the Oxford Ophthalmological Congress in July that year. This was a prized distinction in British ophthalmological circles and the invitation had been the unanimous decision of the Council. (23) The lecture was in memory of Robert Walter Doyne (1857-1916), a British ophthalmologist, who had discovered a rare hereditary form of macular degeneration that led to progressive and irreversible loss of vision. He had founded the Oxford Eye Hospital in 1886, and in 1909 had become the first president of the Oxford Ophthalmological Congress. (24)

The main discussion was to be on 'The Problem of Myopia', because it was 'felt by some that ophthalmologists had been needlessly severe in depriving the myope of all the joys of life that mean so much to him'. (25) Other papers on the programme included the principles underlying the fitting of contact lenses to increase tolerance, hormones and vitamins in ophthalmology, modifications in the technique of corneal grafting, colour photography of the fundus oculi, and 'a profusely illustrated discourse' on plastic surgery of the eyelids by a Budapest professor. A one-eyed aviator, who was 'a first class man in golf, tennis etc'., would also be speaking on his experiences and the problems associated with his disability. (26)

Typically, D.J.W. must have expressed some anxiety about giving the Memorial Lecture because the secretary of the Congress had to convince him that he need have no qualms. They felt sure that he would put up a very fine paper. He was also asked to let them know if he wanted to use lantern slides, which he definitely would have done. His lecture was on 'Night Blindness in Eye Diseases – Suggestions and Speculations', he being the first to describe the condition from the histological viewpoint. (27) The paper was all prepared and he was booked to sail early in May; but his untimely death prevented him from delivering it. Dr. R.C. Meyer of Johannesburg had to read the lecture in his stead, after first paying 'an eloquent tribute in memory of his colleague'. (28)

In his paper D.J.W. laid stress upon the histology of the pigment epithelium, the photochemical changes in the rods and cones, and the significance of vitamin A deficiency as the cause of epidemic night-blindness. His argument hinged on the significance of an intracellular enzyme as the initiator of the changes, which led to the building up of visual purple from vitamin A. He identified a defect of this intracellular enzyme as one of the inborn errors of metabolism. He also suggested that the same enzyme produced pigment pre-natally and metabolized visual purple post-natally. The reported treatment of retinitis pigmentosa by carotene, the precursor of vitamin A, was one indication of the possible chemical processes involved, but this would require further studies. The lecture was published in the *Transactions of the Ophthalmological Society of the United Kingdom*, and was widely regarded as being outstanding. (29)

After D.J.W.'s death, the secretary of the Oxford Ophthalmological Congress sent condolences to Mrs. Wood on behalf of the Master and Council, and the members, saying:

Your husband was held in such high esteem and affection by his colleagues that his loss has been deeply and widely felt. The Doyne Memorial Lecture was listened to with deep interest and respect by 120 Ophthalmic Surgeons from all parts of the Empire, America and the Continent and will be a lasting memorial to a great master in Ophthalmology.(30).

✧

PART 6: 'A MAN'S BEST MONUMENT'

Dr. David James Wood

D.J.W. developed a heart problem fairly early on in life and later on used to take several drops of nitro-glycerine every day as a stimulant. This was a rather dangerous substance, yet it seemed to do the trick for he lived until he was seventy-one. The problem was that he drove himself too hard, refusing to take it easy even when feeling unwell. On the first two days of his final week he continued work as usual even though feeling poorly. He then took to his sickbed for one day, telling a visitor "I am finished". But he did not give up entirely. Even as he lay dying he still had the Doyne lecture on his mind. Rallying to a level of consciousness, he opened his eyes and asked his friend and physician, Dr. Silberbauer, to "please ask Meyer to change line 23 to the following…" Those were his last words. He died of heart failure soon afterwards, on 18 March 1937. (1)

In a tribute to his long-time friend and colleague, Barnard Fuller recalled how the two of them had commenced practice at the end of 1893. Fuller's appointment as Honorary Visiting Surgeon at the New Somerset Hospital had been made soon after D.J.W.'s, and they had both joined the staff of the new Medical School at UCT in 1920. Fuller was Visiting Clinical Lecturer in Surgery specialising in urology, and had been one of the moving spirits in seeing the Medical School established. At the turn of the century he was also the first Medical Officer for Health in Cape Town.

Over those many years the two men had been closely involved with the South African Medical Council and associated bodies. Fuller had retired after thirty-five years at the Hospital and only died in 1946. D.J.W. had stayed on, telling his friend that he would be unhappy if he left. 'He was never more contented than when working at the hospital or in his consulting rooms,' said Fuller, 'and he dreaded the idea of stopping'. (2)

In mid March, 1937, Barnard Fuller had motored D.J.W. up north to a meeting of the S.A.M.C. Committee, and had thought then that his friend was looking very seedy. D.J.W. himself had said sadly that he felt that he was done for. This was his last meeting and he died shortly afterwards. Fuller represented the S.A.M.C. as a pall-bearer at the funeral. He ended his memorial to D.J.W. in the *SAMJ* with these words:

To me, Cape Town will never be the same place without my old colleague, but he has died in harness, full of years and full of honours, without prolonged suffering, and for what more can anyone wish? A modest man, an effective worker, a loyal friend, and an ideal ophthalmologic surgeon, regretted by us all, he has passed. (3)

My grandfather was such an unassuming man that his family did not realise just how admired and famous he was until after his death when they read the obituaries in the newspapers and medical journals. When his estate was wound up it was valued at thirty thousand pounds, a tidy sum of money in those days. The funeral took place in Plumstead Cemetery the day after his death, preceded by a short service at 'Gledsmuir'. He was buried in the family plot EJJ 15. The funeral was attended by the top brass from all the different medical bodies with which he had been associated together with his family and many friends. (4) The Rev. Arthur Blaxall represented the National Council for the Blind and the Athlone School for the Blind, and assisted the Rev. L.W. Liddell at the graveside.

Following D.J.W.'s death, the tributes to him in the local media and medical journals in South Africa and abroad were unanimous in lavishing praise on his distinguished career. In summing up his contribution, the editor of the *British Journal of Ophthalmology* wrote: 'Wood was the doyen of our speciality in South Africa; our Cape Town representative from the start of the Journal, and an ophthalmologist whose reputation extended far beyond the borders of South Africa.'

At home, his Obituary took up pages of the *SAMJ* and has been a mine of information on every aspect of his life. Dr. C. Louis Leipoldt, representing the S.A. Medical Association, spoke of how his humanity, his thoroughness, his indefatigable energy, and his knowledge had rapidly won for him a deserved reputation among the laity. In his profession he was regarded not only as a brilliant eye specialist, but as a most energetic student and scientifically minded man. However, his exceptional modesty meant that many, even in the medical profession, had not realized in what high esteem he had been held across the water. In addressing the local medical fraternity, Leipoldt said:

His passing removes from our ranks a colleague whose life and career should serve as an example and inspiration to all. He gave service ungrudgingly and faithfully to his patients and his students: to the public and the profession he tendered the best, working to the end of his days, and dying – as he would have wished – in harness. He had a fine sense of dignity, and the milk of human kindness never curdled in him. He possessed a keen sense of humour, a thorough knowledge of humanity and a charity that overlooked much. To our Association he gave equally of his best...His criticism was always instructive, pertinent and knowledgeable, and his opinion was therefore received with respect. His death leaves a blank in the profession in the Peninsula, but his life should stimulate those whom he helped in their career as doctors and under whose leadership had the opportunity of studying his methods and his character, while his example should prove to all of us an equal stimulus and inspiration.

In his role as editor of the *SAMJ*, Leipoldt expressed his indebtedness to D.J.W. as a faithful contributor to the journal:

A man's best monument is probably what he has written, as it remains an enduring proof of his work, as well as of his character and ability. The long list of his papers to this Journal and to its predecessors, as well as to the *British Journal of Ophthalmology*, is a worthy record of some of his achievements. (5)

There were many other such tributes by former colleagues and friends following much the same themes. Dr. Barnard Fuller had the final word in expressing his admiration for the man in all his fullness:

Dr. Wood was a very retiring man and never displayed his goods in the window. In his lifetime he did a tremendous amount of free work for poor people. He was a student always. In a quiet and unassuming way he gave his patients, rich and poor alike, all he had culled from his studies. His papers at medical congresses were always worth listening to, and showed careful and systematic research. He was a scientific practitioner in the best sense of the word. (6)

His name lives on in various streets around Cape Town. The Cape Eye Hospital is on the corner of DJ Wood Way in Bellville, and there is also a DJ Wood Terrace at Tygerberg Hospital. We honour his memory as our grandfather, too.

In D.J.W. we see the rare blend of a man of science with a razor-sharp objectivity, and a man of art with a sensual subjectivity. His genius was in harnessing his art to serve his science and exploring his science to heighten his art. The painstaking realism of his paintings, slides, micro-photographs, and sketches enabled him to bring the scientific truths he was exploring to life. In addition to using his professional skills to write and talk about his research, he also wielded his pen, brush, and camera to make a graphic presentation of scientific facts as he unveiled them. As a pioneer in this field, his contributions have left us with a precious legacy, the scope of which is only now being fully realised.

The most endearing quality of D.J.W.'s complex personality was his self-effacing humility. This was born not out of low self-esteem or any other negative qualities, but of a robust respect for the views held by others in his field. This receptiveness made him a true leader in ideas and insights. Ever open to new possibilities and on the lookout for fresh vistas to explore across myriad disciplines, he groomed a generation of young teachers, surgeons and medical artists to carry on the baton. (7)

Above all, D.J.W.'s boundless compassion for people in need of healing gave him the heart that would beat in solidarity with those who feared losing their sight or were blind. This, coupled with his brilliant mind, made him the great surgeon he was, a well-rounded genius ahead of his time, a true humanitarian, a courageous visionary, and last but not least, a lover of all people regardless of colour, creed and class.

D.J.W. shall surely go down as a worthy Ancestor and Elder in the annals of South Africa.

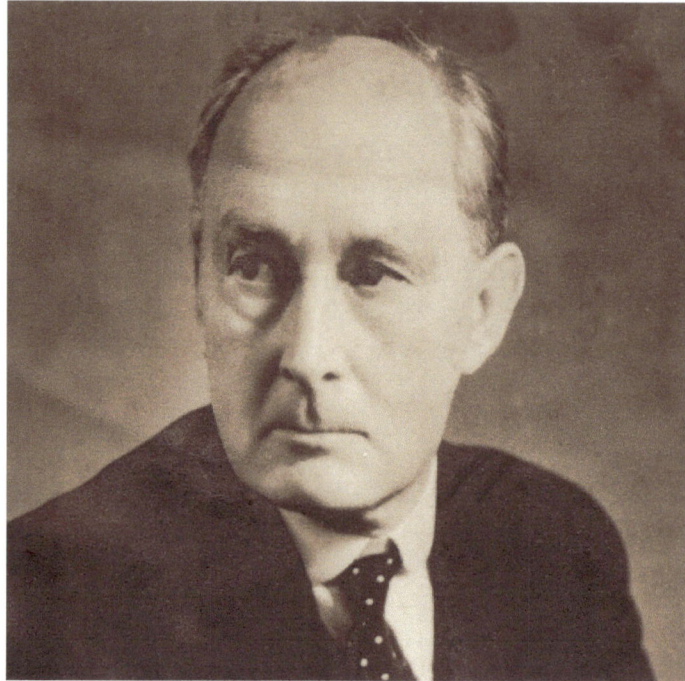

Dr. David James Wood (36)

EPILOGUE
Dr. William Rowland

Past President of the World Blind Union, and Honorary Life President of both Disabled People South Africa and the S.A. National Council for the Blind.

In writing this biography of Dr. David James Wood, South Africa's first ophthalmologist and our first medical specialist, Janet Hodgson has salvaged from oblivion a precious remnant of medical history. Reading her account, we visit in the imagination the bustling streets and leafy suburbs of the Mother City during the first third of the 20th century.

During an extended career in the blindness field I have come to know ophthalmologists as the gentlemen of the medical profession. D.J.W., as he liked to be known, was certainly that and more. I have also found that eye specialists are of two types, those with a singular focus on medical practice and those who show themselves to be men of many parts, men being predominant in this field of medicine. D.J.W. unquestionably belonged to the latter group as is evidenced by his diverse professional pursuits as medical practitioner, avid researcher, prolific author and gifted medical illustrator. He had a love for gardening and for music, and was familiar with the great classics of literature. He somehow found time to make beautiful furniture and he even indulged in motor sport with considerable success.

D.J.W. practised ophthalmology in the centre of Cape Town for well over 40 years. He kept abreast of international trends in his field and pioneered the use in South Africa of early surgical techniques, vaccinations, and many new drugs, all of this before the age of antibiotics, medical electronics, and cryosurgery. In addition to his involvement in various medical associations he was the founding father of the Ophthalmological Society of South Africa and a regular contributor to its publications.

He led an extremely active social life and many famous South Africans of the day crossed his path. He and his wife Constance – herself a woman of note - were friends with the Hennessys, Cloetes and Van der Byls. Olive Schreiner was a neighbour, as was Murray Bisset, the youngest captain of a South African cricket team. C. Louis Leipoldt was a colleague and close friend and famed Cape author, Lawrence G. Green, was also an associate.

Three of the chapters in this book have a particular fascination of their own. In chapter 14 we learn that many of the lepers on Robben Island lost eyesight because of their disease and were patients of D.J.W. He spoke out vehemently in public to draw attention to the appalling conditions prevailing on the island. In the chapter on C. Louis Leipoldt we encounter not only the prominent Cape physician but also the giant of Afrikaans literature and a cookery expert of renown. In the chapter on John Milton we are told that D.J.W. finally resolved the historical debate on the cause of Milton's blindness and his findings throw a revealing light on certain elements in Milton's writing.

The 22 chapters of this thoroughly researched book make for absorbing reading. Janet Hodgson is a meticulous researcher often uncovering unexpected detail and extending her writing into territory off the beaten track. She is the granddaughter of David James Wood and it is an irony of fate that, as she was writing this biography, she was fast losing her eyesight as a result of macular degeneration. That experience is poignantly documented in *Living With Low Vision*. Janet's tenacity of purpose in persisting with her research and writing despite adverse circumstances is greatly to be admired. We thank her for her contribution to historical memory.

✧

Endnotes

Preface

1. OSSA notes that the word 'ophthalmology' comes from Greek roots, *ophthalmos* meaning eye, and *logos* meaning word, thought or discourse. Ophthalmology literally means 'the science of eyes'.

2. Professor Kay de Villiers to Janet Hodgson, 8 June 2009. He held the Helen and Morris Mauerberger Chair of Neurosurgery at the University of Cape Town (UCT). His interest in the history of medicine saw him found the Cape Medical Museum close by the Somerset Hospital, serving as chairman of its Management Committee from 1988 on. He is the author of the three volumes of *Healers, Helpers and Hospitals. A History of Military Medicine in the Anglo-Boer War,* Pretoria: Protea Book House, 2009.

3. Professor Anthony (Tony) Murray was Professor and Head of the Department of Ophthalmology at UCT from 1985 to 2006.

Chapter 1

1. The information in this chapter and the next is taken from D.J.W.'s 'A Retrospect', and from his mother, Christina Wood's handwritten notebooks, which are not always easy to decipher.

Chapter 2

1. Burgess were upper class inhabitants of a town or borough, particularly if they had full municipal rights. This would include Members of Parliament and magistrates.

2. The Royal High School of Edinburgh is said to be the 18th oldest school in the world. In 1505 it was the first in Britain to be designated a high school.

Chapter 3

1. Personal recollections are taken from D.J.W.'s 'A Retrospect'.

2. See http://en.wikipedia.org/wiki/Argyll_Robertson_ pupils.

3. I am indebted to Dr. Gideon du Plessis for this information: 'The Life and Times of D.J.Wood – Part 1', 28th D.J.Wood Memorial Lecture, February 2010, *SA Ophthalmology Journal,* 8 (2), Autumn 2013, p.22.

4. See: www.moorfields.nhs.uk/;http://en.wikipedia.org/wiki/Moorfields.

5. Retrieved from http://en.wikipedia.org/wiki/Moorfields_Eye_Hospital_NHS_Foundation_Trust.

6. Ibid.

7. Robert Marcus Gunn (1850-1909) received his medical training in Scotland. A Fellow of the Royal College of Surgeons, he was appointed surgeon at Moorfields in 1888. He later took on other prestigious hospital appointments and became Vice-President, and then President, of the Ophthalmological Section of the British Medical Association in 1906. His particular contribution was 'Gunn's sign and the Marcus Gunn pupil'. He lectured in Vienna before coming to Moorfields and used this experience to introduce the principles of sterility in surgery as devised by Dr. John Lister.

8. John Couper (1835-1918) was also a Scotsman. His medical training included anatomy, physiology and operative surgery. This led him to becoming Professor in these disciplines in the London Hospital. He became interested in ophthalmology and, together with A. Stanford Morton, developed a 'magazine ophthalmoscope, which facilitated the measurement not only of errors of refraction but of degrees of astigmatism'. He was among the last of the general surgeons to practice ophthalmology, giving a special course of lectures on diseases of the eye at his hospital: Plarr's Lives of the Fellows Online.

9. Arthur Quarry Silcock (1855-1904), an Englishman, had a meteoric career in the Medical Department of University College, London. He then became Lecturer in Pathology at St. Mary's Hospital as well as instructor in operative surgery. Early on he also became interested in ophthalmology. When he was appointed a full surgeon at Moorfields, he was the only staff member who was also surgeon at a General Hospital and Medical School. His wide medical and surgical knowledge contributed to his success with ophthalmic work. He is remembered for the ophthalmic needle holder: Plarr's Lives of the Fellows Online.

10. Edward Nettleship (1845-1913) was also English. Prior to specializing in ophthalmology, he studied veterinary medicine and dermatology. He worked at the London Hospital and Moorfields before going on to be ophthalmic surgeon and lecturer at St. Thomas' Hospital, London. He is remembered for his work with hereditary eye disorders, making 'important contributions in the research of ocular albinism, retinitis pigmentosa and hereditary night blindness'. The Nettleship Medal of the British Ophthalmological Society was created in his honour: Plarr's Lives of the Fellows Online; http://en.wikipedia.org/wiki/Edward_Nettleship.

11. See http://www.whonamedit.com/doctor.cfm/983.html.

12. Du Plessis, 2013, pp.22-23.

Chapter 4

1. Waren Tay (often misspelt Warren) (1843-1027), a Yorkshireman, studied medicine at London Hospital. He then held positions in skin diseases at Blackfriars and in a children's hospital, becoming a member of the Royal College of Surgeons. He worked with Edward Nettleship under Jonathan Hutchinson at Moorfields, and eventually became senior surgeon. He was a founding member of the British Ophthalmological Society, and was the first to describe the red spot on the retina of the eye, known as Tay-Sachs disease, in Volume I of their journal. While at Moorfields during 1874-5, he was also 'the first to describe the condition that consists of small white or yellow dots in the choroids around the macula in the eye. These are the manifestations of senile macular degeneration', sometimes referred to as 'Hutchinson's disease' or 'Tay's choroiditis': whonamedit.com/doctor.cfm/474.html; http://en.wikipedia.org/wiki/Waren_Tay. Tay suffered from glaucoma and was blind in one eye. A keen cyclist he was also known as 'a walking encyclopaedia of medicine'. See also http://www.whonamedit.com/doctor.cfm.474.html.

2. Sir John Tweedy (1849-1924), a Fellow of the College of Surgeons, came from Stockton-on-Tees. He started as a clinical assistant at Moorfields in 1873, became an assistant surgeon in 1884, and then a full surgeon. He also took an editorial post at *The Lancet* for a time. In 1886 he became Professor of Ophthalmic Medicine and Surgery at University College, London.

3. William Lang (1852-1937) was another Fellow of the Royal College of Surgeons. As a skilled surgeon and eye specialist, he published numerous papers regarding diseases of the eye. He is reputed to have taken control of the body of an American medium and psychic healer, George Chapman, who performed psychic surgery on patients ten years after Lang's death.

4. Dr. E. Barnard Fuller, 'Obituary', *SAMJ,* 10 April 1937, p. 248.

5. 'The Presentation to Dr. D.J. Wood', *SAMJ*, December 1895, p.226.

6. Jane Waterston came to South Africa with Dr. James Stewart, the Scottish missionary, when he became principal of Lovedale College in the Eastern Cape. She founded the Girl's Institution there. In 1874 she returned to England and was one of the first to train as a doctor at the London School of Medicine for Women. After graduating she worked briefly in Nyasaland before settling at the Cape in 1887, where she started the first maternity service. She was known for her work among the poor, providing free nursing and medicine.

7. J. Foster, F.R.C.S. to S. Goldwyn, Leeds, 12 May 1936.

Chapter 5

1. Helen Robinson, *Beyond the City Limits. People and Property at Wynberg, 1795-1927*, Cape Town: Juta & Co., 1998, pp.19, 46, 75. See also http://ancestry24.com/history-of-plumstead/.

2. Colonel Richard George Southey's (1844-1909) final appointment was as Colonial Military Secretary from 1903 to 1904. He wrote a clause in his will that no flats were to be built below the railway line. Many of the streets in the area have Devon names, in memory of his home county. His house, 'Southfields', later became St. Michael's Orphanage.

3. Murray Bisset (1876-1931) also served in the South African War. His record as the youngest Test cricket captain was only beaten in 1957 when Ian Craig captained Australia.

4. Robinson, 1998, pp.162-163, 209.

Chapter 6

'1. I am greatly indebted to Derek Stuart-Findlay who went to great trouble in doing research for this section, and especially D.J.W.'s role in winning the 1912 trial run to Caledon and back : 'The Siddeley Cup - admission to the Sanatorium', *The Crankhandle Chronicle*. June 2013, pp.10-11.

2. Hennessy's Quad was imported by W.M. Jenkins, manager of Garlicks Cycle Supply, part of the Garlicks Department Store in St. George's Street.

His second car was a Deauville. The story is related by William Andrew

Kerkham in his Reminscences (1990): Andrew Summers Kerkham

(transcriber and editor), 2005, ch.7, 'Transport':

http://freepages.genealogy.rootsweb.amcestry.com/-kerkham/wak.htm.

3. Lawrence G. Green, *I Heard The Old Men Say*, Cape Town: Howard Timmins, 1964, pp.278-29 – based on a report in the *Cape Argus*, March 1899.

4. Lawrence G. Green, *Tavern of the Seas*, Cape Town: Howard Timmins, 1947, pp.78-79.

5. Kerkham, (1990) 2005, ch.7, 'Transport'.

6. Green, 1964, p.283.

7. In August 1905, the Johannesburg to Cape Town run was done in 10 days: Green, 1947, pp.78-79.

8. Green, 1964, p.280.

9. The Clement-Talbots were initially imported from France to North Kensington, London. They were known as Talbots after 1903 and the first British made model appeared in 1906: Stuart-Findley to Hodgson, 22 March 2013.

10. Born in 1866, John Davenport Siddeley promoted pneumatic tyres for bicycles in England during the 1890s and went on to experiment with them on motor vehicles. He founded Siddeley Autocars in 1902, building English bodies on imported Peugeot mechanicals. In 1905 the company merged with Wolseley to produce the Wolseley-Siddeley. In 1909, Siddeley took over the Deasy Motor Co. to make Siddeley-Deasy cars. Their slogan was 'Silent as the Sphinx': Stuart-Findley to Hodgson, 24 March 2013; and his article in *The Crankhandle Chronicle*, June 2013.

11. All information on the Siddeley Cup was provided by Derek Stuart-Findley, 21 March 2013. The first Siddeley Cup trial took place on 20 February 1909 with a tie for first place between C. Mills and C.F. Spilhaus.

12. The Pass cost seven thousand pounds to make but the Secretary of State in London begrudged the money and Cape Town merchants had to come to the rescue: Lawrence G. Green, *In the Land of the Afternoon*, Cape Town: Howard Timmins, 1949, p.37.

13. Dr. W. Darley-Hartley, 'The Mineral Waters of Caledon', read as a paper at the East London Medical Congress, 1908, and G.W.B. Daniell, abstract of a paper read at the Cape Town Medical Congress, 1893, *SAMJ*, 23 November 1940, pp.437-42. The Caledon Baths complex was burnt down in 1946 and the new hotel was not built until 1990.

14. The minutes of the Automobile Club of South Africa's meetings are missing for this period, but fortunately they started a monthly magazine in August 1912 called *Motoring in South Africa*, from which Stuart-Findlay obtained this information: Stuart-Findley to Hodgson, 26 March 2013.

15. Stuart-Findlay to Hodgson, 24 March 2013.

16. The ramifications of Siddeley's subsequent mergers with Vickers and then Sir Thomas (Tommy) Sopwith are too complex to follow, but he was knighted for his work in developing the aircraft industry in 1932, and became Baron Kenilworth that same year. He died in 1956 at the age of 90: Stuart-Findlay to Hodgson, 22 and 24 March 2013.

17. R.L.H. Townsend, 'The Development of Ophthalmology in Cape Town', unpublished MS filed in the Department of Ophthalmology, UCT, March 1962.

18. Robinson, 1998, ch.4; See also http://www.atlanticrail.co.za/stations_history.php.

19. 'Mr Hansom's Patent Safety Cab' had first been imported by Sir Robert Stanford in 1849.

20. Lawrence G. Green, *So Few Are Free*, Cape Town: Howard Timmins, 1946, pp.15-16.

21. The first tram line, opened in 1897, ran as far as Camp Street; but the system was soon extended across Cape Town: Kerkham, 2005, ch.7, 'Transport'.

22. The cab ride from Cape Town to Wynberg took one hour and 10 minutes: Lawrence G. Green, *Secrets of Africa*, London: Stanley Paul, 1938, pp.137-142. For further information on cabs see Green, 1946, pp.15-16; 1947, p.6; and 1964, pp.278-281; Eric Rosenthal, *Fish Horns and Hansom Cabs. Life in Victorian Cape Town*, Cape Town: Ad Donker, 1977.

Chapter 7

1. J.L. van Selm, 'Children with Learning Disabilities', D.J. Wood Memorial Lecture, April 1979.

2. For further information: www.thefreedictionary.com/micrograph; http://www.rieggat.com/phothistory/history/micro_ph.htm.

3. See for example D.J. Wood. 'Observations on the Human Retina' with 8 photographs of sections on glass plates; and 'Inflammatory Diseases of the Eye Caused by Gout' with 7 large photographs of sections on glass plates, *BJO*, XIX July 1935, pp.369-377, and XX, September 1936, pp.510-519.

4. See http://www.capetownpartnership.co.za/programmes/public-space-for-public-life/church-square/.

Chapter 8

1. It was after an exhibition of his scenic paintings in Durban that he painted a portrait of a ricksha boy, subsequently exhibited at the Paris Salon and the Royal Academy, London.

2. Much of the information on Tinus de Jongh is drawn from Esme Berman, *Art and Artists of South Africa*, Cape Town: A.A. Balkema, 1983, pp.76-77.

3. Berman, 1983, p.76.

4. For information on medical illustrations: http://en.wikipedia.org/wiki/ Medical_illustrator.

5. Pieter van der Bijl, 'Medical Art – A brief general overview, and its development in South Africa', student paper for *SAMJFoRUM*, SAMJ, 91 (12), December 2001.

6. Max Brodel, an artist who came from Leipzig in the late 1890s, founded the Department of Applied Medical Art at John Hopkins School of Medicine in Baltimore in 1911, the first such institution in the world: http://en.wikipedia.org/ wiki/Medcial_Illustrator.

7. A set of black and white photographs of eyes mounted on cardboard have been lost over the years.

Chapter 9

1. This chapter is largely based on family reminiscences.

2. See *Women of South Africa,* 1913, Cape Town: Scribes Publishing.

3. Lewis Simms later became Braam's Butchery and then Sam's Meat Centre. It was connected through an inter-leading passage to the grocery section of Fletcher and Cartwright next door in Longmarket Street, and one could walk through from one shop to the other: Kerkham, 2005, ch.9, 'Shops and Foods'.

4. Green, 1947, pp.190-200. The first 'Fair and Show' of the Cape Flats Farmers' Association was held in the Claremont Town Hall on 9 April 1892 as a way of proving the fertility of the area.

Chapter 10

1. Vivian Bickford-Smith, Elizabeth van Heyningen, Nigel Worden, *Cape Town in the Twentieth Century,* Cape Town: David Philip, 1999, p.32.

2. T.R.H. Davenport, *South Africa. A Modern History*, 2nd ed., Johannesburg: Macmillan South Africa, 1978, pp.173-5.

3. Thelma Gutsche, *No Ordinary Woman. The Life and Times of Florence Phillips*, Cape Town: Howard Timmins, 1966, pp.307-9, 323-4, 330.

4. Gutsche, 1966, pp. 186-7, 192-7.

5. Bickford-Smith et al, 1999, p.30.

6. Bickford-Smith et al, 1999, pp.48-9.

7. Helen Robinson, *Beyond the City Limits. People and Property at Wynberg*, 1795-1927, Cape Town: Juta & Co., 1998, pp.209, 223-4.

8. Robinson, 1998, p.215.

9. Robinson, 1998, pp. 209, 212-213, 226-8.

Chapter 11

1. G.D. Nel, *Jerseys in Southern Africa*, Cape Town: Tafelberg 1968, pp.28-9.

2. The Rev. John R. de Lingen-Kilburn, to give him his full name, was born in Russia but came from a line of Scottish Presbyterian ministers. Despite being raised in a strictly Reformed Calvanist ethos, he morphed into an ardent Indophile and student of Hinduism. I am indebted to the Rev. Jayant Kothare for information on De Lingen.

3. *The Cape Times*, 16 August 1947.

Chapter 12

1. Editor, 'Obituary', *SAMJ*, XI (7), 10 April 1937, p. 249.

2. I am indebted to Dr. Gideon du Plessis for information on the inaugural symphony concert. His research ended up at the Royal College of Music in London, where they traced the original programme. The concertmaster was the violinist Ellie Marx: Du Plessis to Hodgson, 22 July 2013.

3. A.D.N. Murray, 'Survival with Excellence: Ophtalmology Today and in the Future', Inaugural Lecture as Helen and Morris Mauerberger Professor of the Department of Opthalmology, UCT, New Series no.122, 3 September 1986, pp.2-3. Professor Murray has placed historic photographs and newspaper cuttings of early cataract surgery in the Ophthalmology Department library at the Groote Schuur Medical School.

4. Dr C.M. Murray, 'Obituary', *SAMJ*, XI (7), 10 April 1937, p.247.

5. This testimony was sent to my father by my cousin, Dr. Robin Newbery, then practising in King William's Town. Both Charles Woolley's father and grandfather had served in the navy.

6. Letter in Wood Papers, 20 November 1928.

7. *Cape Argus*, 18 March 1937.

8. See Jackie Loos, 'Light in a dark corner of apartheid', *Cape Argus*, 13 December 2000, p.17, from which some of this account is taken. The article is accompanied by a photograph of the boy from Venda learning arithmetic on a Taylor Frame in 1936. The original material is found in A.W. Blaxall, *Ten Cameos from Darkest Africa*, Lovedale: Lovedale Press 1937. After a geyser burst in 1928, two sections of the school were badly damaged by fire. The school was moved to a permanent home in Kasselsvlei Road, Bellville, in 1941.

9. Arthur Blaxall, who suffered from a collapsed lung, later moved to the Transvaal but never stopped working for the underprivileged. His religious beliefs, pacifism and efforts to promote inter-racial reconciliation led to his arrest in 1963. He was found guilty of aiding the ANC and PAC under the Suppression of Communism Act but was paroled after one night in prison. He returned to Britain where he died in 1970.

10. Blaxall, 1937, p.31.

11. Ibid., pp.17-18.

12. Correspondence from various members of the Government and Services in the Wood Papers.

Chapter 13

1. J.H. Louw, *In the Shadow of Table Mountain. A history of the University of Cape Town Medical School and its associated teaching hospitals up to 1950, with glimpses of the future*, Cape Town: Struik Publishing, 1969, p.10.

2. Work on the Shipley Pavilion was commenced in 1914, and was named in memory of Mr. Joseph Shipley, whose estate bequeathed the funds. Mr. and Mrs. Brown added a donation of one thousand pounds to equip and furnish the building. It was opened by Sir Frederic de Waal.

3. Louw, 1969, p.176.

4. Ibid.

5. J.L. van Selm, 1979, p.88.

6. Townsend, 1962, pp. 3-5.

7. Louw, 1969, p.246.

8. Murray, 1986, p.2.

9. See http//en.wikipedia.org/wiki/Slit_Lamp.

10. Townsend, 1962, p.8.

11. Dr. J.S. du Toit, 'Obituary', *SAMJ, XI* (7), 10 April 1937, p.249.

12. Townsend, 1962, pp.4-5.

13. Dr. du Toit was on the UCT Council for many years. Having been born and brought up in Worcester, he also served their School for the Blind for twenty-one years. Dr. Sichel had an equally distinguished career. This included being President of the Medical Association of S.A. (1945-51), and of the British Medical Association (1951-2).

14. J.L. Van Selm, 'Obituary: R.L.H. Townsend', n.d.

Chapter 14

1. Harriet Deacon, 'The Medical Institutions on Robben Island', in Harriet Deacon (ed.), *The Island. A History of Robben Island, 1488-1990*, Cape Town and University of the Western Cape: David Philip and Mayibuye Books, pp.57-75. See also Nigel Penn, Harriet Deacon, Neville Alexander, *Robben Island: The Politics of Rock and Sand*, University of Cape Town, 1992.

2. George Newman, *Prize Essays on Leprosy*, London: The Society, 1895, p.194.

3. Lawrence G. Green, *Grow Lovely, Growing Old*, Cape Town: Howard Timmins, 1951, p.257. Green regularly sailed over to the island in his boat and so was familiar with the conditions of the lepers.

4. Barbara Hutton, *Robben Island. Symbol of Resistance*, Johannesburg and Cape Town: SACHED and Mayibuye Books, 1994, pp.29-32.

5. Green, 1946, p.40.

6. See http://rarediseases.about.com/cs/infectiousdisease/a/07/1203.htm.

7. 'Nurses of Robben Island': http://ancestry24.com/nurses-of-robben-island/.

8. The All Saints sisters had come from St. Alban's in England in 1876. Their Mother House in Cape Town was at St. Michael's Home in Kloof Street. For the religious life of the lepers and their daily lives see the Rev. W.U. Watkins, Chaplain, 'Robben Island', in A.M.S, Gibson, *Sketches of Church Work and Life in the Diocese of Capetown*, Cape Town: S.A. Electric Printing and Publishing, 1900, Chapter V.

9. Green, 1951, p.257.

10. Green, 1946, p.41.

11. For the full report: 'The Eye Complications of Leprosy', *SAMR*, XI, 28 June 1913, pp.245-6.

12. D.J. Wood, 'Ocular Leprosy', *BJO*, VIII, January 1925, pp.1-4.

13. Before then up to 1000 lepers had lived on the island, together with 500 'lunatics', around 500 officials and their families, and 100 convicts: Green 1946, p.39.

Chapter 15

1. Editorial, 'Obituary', *SAMJ*, 1937.

2. Murray, 1937, p.247.

3. I am indebted to Richard Keeler, for this information from an Obituary of D.J.W. He is Hon. Curator of the Royal College of Ophthalmologists, and Hon. Archivist of the Moorfields Alumni Association.

4. J.C. de Villiers, 2009.

5. D.J.Wood, 'The Treatment of Bacterial Diseases by Vaccines', an inaugural Presidential address to the C.G.H. (Western) Branch of the B.M.A., *SAMR*, IV (6), 10 April 1906, p.89.

6. Dr. E. Barnard Fuller, 'Obituary', *SAMJ*, XI (7), 10 April 1937, p.248.

7. Wood, 1906, pp.85-91.

8. Barnard Fuller, 1937, p.248.

9. J.S. du Toit, 'Obituary', *SAMJ*, XI (7), 10 April 1937, p.249.

10. D.J. Wood, 'Correspondence – Dr. Wood and the District Surgeons' Association', *SAMR*, June 1903.

11. *SAMR*, XII, June 1914, pp.192-4.

Chapter 16

1. In 2010, Professor de Villiers was awarded the Simon van der Stel Gold Medal by Heritage South Africa for 'his efforts in establishing the Cape Medical Museum, and for his historical research on the medical aspects of the Anglo Boer War'.

2. On the appointment of its first curator in 1982 it was proclaimed a Provincial Museum, and opened in the New Somerset Hospital four years later. In 1992, after two moves, it finally found its present home off Portswood Road in the Old City Hospital Complex, Green Point.

3. Small collections were given by the Western Branch of the S.A. Medical Association, Professor Jannie Louw, Professor Bromilow Downing and Professor de Villiers: De Villiers to Hodgson, 7 June 2009.

4. The most valuable item historically is a medicine chest, which was in the Atherstone family from 1815. Complete with original bottles and medicines, it belonged to Dr. John Atherstone, who practised in Grahamstown until 1850. It was then passed on to his son, Guy, who, in 1847, was the first doctor in South Africa to use ether as an anaesthetic.

5. This information is taken from an undated newspaper report of an interview with Mrs. Anista Keyser, a former history teacher who became the first curator of the museum.

6. Alarik Frithiof Homgren (1831-1897), a Swedish physiologist, developed the test in response to a railway accident in which the engineer was suspected of being colour-blind. In 1879 it became the standardized test for colour-blindness (or colour vision deficiency).

7. Homgren's theory was that there are three sets of colour perceiving elements in the retina, and a defect in one of these elements causes a variety of colour-blindness. In his test a patient is required to match the coloured skeins of wool correctly under normal lighting conditions. See for example http://www.psych.utoronto.ca/museum/holmgren.htm; http://whonamedit.com/synd.cfm/2515.html.

8. This paper was published with a photograph and 8 Scotoma chart diagrams, in *SAMJ*, X (16), August 1936, pp.580-583.

9. The Adler Museum of Medicine at the University of the Witwatersrand Medical School houses an historic ophthalmic section but to my knowledge does not contain any of D.J.W.'s material.

10. Stuart-Findlay, 2013, pp.10-11. The line up is identified as D. Wood's Talbot, A. Hennessy's Standard, P.White's Napier, two Rovers (one possibly driven by C. Garlick), W. Long's Sunbeam, J.W. Jagger's Delaunay-Belleville, and a Panhard.

Chapter 17

1. D.J. Wood, 'An Ophthalmological Society' together with Draft Rules,

22 December 1930, *Journal of the Medical Association of S.A. (B.M.A,) (JMASA)*, V (1), 10 January 1931, pp.29-30, with an explanatory letter following in *JMASA*, V (2), p.30.

2. The five committee members selected were Drs. Meyer, Seale, Verwey, Wilson and Wood.

3. Leading Article, 'An Ophthalmological Society', *JMASA*, V (1), 10 January 1931.

4. Inaugural Address, *JMASA*, V (2), pp.816-817. See also Van Selm, 1979, pp.88-9.

5. Hulke was renowned as a geologist, specialising in collecting fossils. He was made Fellow of the Royal Society for his work on the eyes of lower animals, chiefly those of reptiles.

6. L. Staz, 'Randon Reminscences in the 40 years lifetime of the Ophthalmological Society of South Africa', published by OSSA, Johannesburg, n.d., pp.43-4.

7. See numerous obituaries.

8. See Appendix 5 for a list of those who have given the D.J.Wood Memorial Lectures between 1976 and 2013. Unfortunately, no record has been kept of their topics. A number of ophthalmologists have helped piece together the available information but it is sadly incomplete and I apologise for any errors.

Chapter 18

1. *SAMJ*, I, March 1984, p. 226.

2. 'The Glands of the Ciliary Body', *SAMJ*, I, April 1894, pp. 246-7.

3. The ciliary body is a circular structure just behind the iris composed of the ciliary muscle and ciliary processes, which attach to the lens. The ciliary processes secrete the aqueous humour, the clear fluid between the lens and the cornea, and the ciliary muscle modifies focus by changing the dhape of the lens.

4. 'Fluorescein', and 'Errors of Refraction and Epilepsy', *SAMJ*, II, April 1894, pp.22-3.

5. 'Blinding of the Retina from Direct Sunlight', *SAMJ*, II, June 1894, p.57.

6. 'Detachment of the Retina', *JMASA*, II, October 1928, pp.513-7.

7.'Infective Ulceration of the Cornea', *SAMJ*, II, July 1894, pp.73-4.

8. 'Ophthalmic Notes. Miscellaneous Reports from other countries compared with local experiences', *S*AMJ, III, May 1895, pp.18-19.

9. 'A Case of Hereditary Specific Iritis in a Young Child', SAMJ, III part 2, July 1895, p.68.

10. 'Two Cases of Diseases of the Eye – Ciliary Staphyloma and Opthelmia Neonatorium', *SAMJ*, IV part 3, July 1896, p, 63.

11. 'Injuries and Common Diseases of the Eye', *SAMR*, XX, October 1922, pp. 390-8.

12. 'Some Cases of Retinal Disease Associated with Streptococcic Infection', *SAMR*, XXII, 10 October 1925, pp.431-5. The oldest patient was 34 and four were under 20.

13. 'The Co-ordimeter of Prof. Ness', *SAMR*, XXIII, 13 June 1925, pp.235-6.

14. 'The Optic Nerve Aspect of the Diagnosis of Intra-Cranial Tumours', *SAMR*, XIII, 14 November 1925, pp.475-8.

15. 'The Resistance of the Lamina Cribosa as a Factor in Glaucoma', *JMASA*, V (8), 25 April 1931, pp.251-4.

16. 'A Case of Supra-stellar Meningioma', *SAMJ*, X (16), 22 August 1936, pp.580-3.

17. 'Staining of the Cornea by Blood-pigment', *SAMJ*, IX (5), March 1935, pp.2-4.

18. 'Some Fundus Conditions', *JMASA*, V (24), 26 December 1931, pp.817-8.

19. 'Clinical Notes. Avulsion of an Eye', *SAMJ*, X (17), 12 September 1936, p.611.

20. 'Trachoma Problems', *SAMJ*, X (17), 26 September 1936, pp.629-31.

Chapter 19

1. For further information on Leipoldt and his medical career see J.C. Kannemeyer, **Leipoldt,** *'n Lewensverhaal*, Cape Town: Tafelberg, 1999, chapter 15, 'Pediater, Pedagoog en die Mediese Vereneging'; BC 94, The Louis Leipoldt Papers, Manuscripts and Archives, University of Cape Town Libraries, list compiled by Etaine Eberhard, 1981; Lawrence G. Green, *On Wings of Fire*, Cape Town: Howard Timmins, 1967, pp. 151-162.

2. Lawrence G. Green, *I Heard the Old Men Say*, Cape Town: Howard Timmins, 1964, p.110.

3. His journal offices were in the Southern Life building in St. George's Street, Cape Town. In 1936 he moved to Medical House in Wale Street. The Afrikaans title to the journal was added in 1932.

4. J.H. Louw, 'Leipoldt the paediatrician', *Suid-Afrikaanse Mediese Tydskrif (SAMJ)*, 6 December 1980, p. 505.

5. Louw, 1980. p.500.

6. All the following quotations, remarks and reminiscences are taken from the obituary written by the Editor, Dr. C. Louis Leipoldt, *SAMJ*, 10 April 1937, pp.248-9.

7. Editorial Leader, *SAMJ*, XI (7), 10 April 1937.

Chapter 20

1. All references are taken from 'The Blindness of John Milton', a monograph of 12 pages reprinted from the *SAMJ*, 23 November 1935, Cape Town: Cape Times.

Chapter 21

1. Christine A. Iacobuzio-Donohue (an anatomical pathologist) and Norman Baker (medical photographer) (eds.), *Hidden Beauty: Exploring the Aesthetics of Medical Science*, Atglen, Lancaster. Pennsylvania: Schiffer Publications, 2013.

2. The *BJO* is a peer-reviewed medical journal covering all aspects of ophthalmology. It was founded in 1917 by the amalgamation of the Royal London (Moorfields) Ophthalmological Reports with the Ophthalmoscope and Opthalmological Record.

3. 'Obituary, D.J. Wood', *BJO*, XXI, June 1937, pp.332-3.

4. 'Obituary, D.J. Wood', *BJO*, 1937. I am indebted to Richard Keeler for his archival research in London.

5. 'Three Cases of Total Removal of Iris', *BJO*, IV, September 1920, pp.412-3.

6. 'Detached Retina', *BJO*, IV, September 1920, pp.413-5.

7. 'Accommodative Failure in Malaria and Influenza', *BJO*, IV, September 1920, pp. 415-6.

8. 'Ocular Leprosy', *BJO*, VIII, January 1925, pp.1-4.

9. 'Hyatid cysts of the Orbit', *BJO*, VIII, January 1925, pp.4-6. He attributed the recovery of vision to 'the absence of degenerative changes in the nerves, which was in agreement with the absence of fundus changes'.

10. 'Conjunctival Pemphigus', *BJO*, V. March 1921, pp.123-4. The simple treatment involved saline irrigation, zinc sulphate drops, and a little white Vaseline at night. Complete occlusion of both eyes was required whenever the disease seemed to be advancing.

11. 'Onyx of Long Duration', *BJO*, VI, October 1922, p.458.

12. 'Intra-Ocular Cysticercus', *BJO*, VI, October 1922, pp.459-61.

13. 'Two Cases of Non-Traumatic Cysts of the Interior Chamber', *BJO*, IX, September 1925, pp.450-4.

14. 'A Case of Sympathetic Ophthalmitis', *BJO*, XI, May 1927, pp.217-224.

15. 'Two Cases of Sympathetic Ophthalmitis', *BJO*, XIV, June 1930, pp.291-7.

16. 'Calcium Deficiency in the Blood with Reference to Spring Catarrh and Malignant Myopia', *BJO*, XI, May 1927, pp.224-230; Letter on 'Calcium Deficiencies', *BJO*, XI, August 1927, p.415.

17. 'Melanosis of the Iris and New Formation of a Hyaline Membrane on its Surface', *BJO*, March 1928, pp.143-6.

18. 'A Suggestion as to the Cause of Glaucoma Following Thrombosis of the Retinal Vein', *BJO,* XVI, July 1932, pp.423-4.

19. 'An Unusual Result following Traumatic Irido-Cyclitis', *BJO*, XVI, September 1932, pp.546-8.

20. 'A Case of Congenital Cataract Showing Unusual features', *BJO*, XVII, March 1933, pp.158-161.

21. 'Observations on the Human Retina', *BJO*, XIX, July 1935, pp.369-377.

22. 'Inflammatory Disease in the Eye Caused by Gout', *BJO*, XX, September 1936, pp. 510-9.

23. F.A. Anderson, Secretary and Treasurer of the Oxford Ophthalmological Congress to Dr. Wood, 21 November 1936; *The Cape Times*, 19 March 1937.

24. In 1899 Doyne discovered the disorder that became known as 'Doyne's honeycomb choroiditis'. It has also been called 'macular drusen', 'malattia leventinese', 'dominant radial drusen', and 'Doyne honeycomb retinal dystrophy'. He was also the first to describe angloid streaks, a disorder that affects Bruch's membrane: The Ophthalmology Hall of Fame — http://www.mrcophth.com/ophthalmologyhalloffame/doyne.html.

25. Anderson to Wood, 28 December 1936.

26. *Transactions of the Ophthalmological Society of the United Kingdom, LVII, part 2, Session 1937*, London: J. and A. Churchill Ltd., Illustrated version, 1938 – 'Correspondence', *BJO*, XXII (6), June 1938, p.381.

27. Van Selm, 1979, p.87.

28. 'Night Blindness', Report on the Doyne Memorial Lecture by Dr. D.J. Wood, Oxford Ophthalmological Congress, *The British Medical Journal*, 17 July 1937, p.132. The summarised contents of the paper are taken from this report.

29. I am indebted to the Rev. Jayant Kothare for his assistance in editing this chapter.

30. Anderson to Mrs. Wood, 15 July 1937.

PART 6

1. Van Selm, 1979, p.87.

2. Dr. E. Barnard Fuller, 'Obituary', *SAMJ*, XI (7), 10 April 1937, p.247.

3. Barnard Fuller, 1937, p.248.

4. The pall bearers were Sir Carruthers Beattie (University of Cape Town), Dr. T.L. Sandes (Medical Association of South Africa), Professor A.W. Falconer (Cape Town University Medical School), Dr. E. Barnard Fuller (South African Medical Council), Dr. J.S. du Toit (Ophthalmological Society of South Africa), Dr. A.W. Sichel, Dr. A. Simpson Wells, Dr. J. Luckoff, and Dr. A.J. Moffat: Editorial, 'Obituary, Dr. Wood', *SAMJ*, XI (7), 10 April 1937, p.247.

5. Leipoldt's quotations are taken from the editorial, *SAMJ*, XI (7), 10 April 1937. See also *Cape Argus*, 18 March 1937.

6. Dr. E. Barnard Fuller, *The Cape Times*, 19 March 1937.

7. I am indebted to the Rev. Jayant Kothare for his critical insights, editorial assistance, proofreading and invaluable contributions regarding the life and work of my grandfather.

Sources

Dr. D.J. Wood's Writing in Wood Family Papers

D.J. Wood, M.B., C.M. Edin., 'Sheet IV – Intoxicants and Narcotics, Drainage and Ventilation, etc.', *Handbook to Illustrations of Human Anatomy, Physiology, and Hygiene*, London: Ruddiman Johnston & Co., n.d., 31 pages (inscribed by the author, November 12th 1889).

D.J. Wood, 'A Retrospect', 10 pages unpublished and undated (c1935).

D.J. Wood, 'The Treatment of Bacterial Diseases by Vaccines', an Inaugural Presidential Address to the Cape of Good Hope (Western) Branch of the British Medical Association, *The South African Medical Record*, IV (6), April 10, 1906, pp.85-91.

D.J. Wood, 'The Blindness of John Milton', monograph reprinted from *South African Medical Journal*, November 23, 1935.

D.J. Wood, Ophthalmological and Clinical Notes, Correspondence, and numerous Articles, including addresses and lectures he had given at various conferences and meetings, printed in *The South African Medical Record, The South African Medical Journal – S.A. Tydskrif vir Geneeskunde, The Journal of the Medical Association of S.A. (B.M.A.), The British Journal of Ophthalmology*, between 1894 and 1936.

Wood Family Papers

Wood Family Papers, held by Julie M. Hodgson:

- Julie M. Hodgson, 'Wood Family Tree'.

- David Wood's birth certificate and passport.

- Photographs of David and Constance Wood, and some family pictures.

- Obituaries: Dr. D.J. Wood – Editor (Dr. C. Louis Leipoldt), Dr. C.M. Murray, Dr. E. Barnard Fuller, Dr. J.S. du Toit – *S. A. Medical Journal/S.A. Tydskrif vir Geneeskunde*, XI (7), April 10, 1937, Editorial and pp.246-249; *British Journal of Ophthalmology*, XXI (6), June 1937, pp.332-3; letter from Hon. Secretary, Oxford Ophthalmological Society to Mrs. Wood, 15 July 1937; *Cape Argus*, 18 March 1937; *Cape Times*, 19 March 1937.

- *Cape Times*, 'Funeral of Mrs. D.J.Wood', 16 August 1943.

- A collection of notebooks with Scottish family and historical information written by Christine Smith Wood (D.J.W.'s mother).

- D.J. Wood, 'A Retrospect', the article on the blindness of John Milton, 1935, and *Handbook on Human Anatomy, Physiology, and Hygiene*, 1889.

- Correspondence from various defence forces relating to D.J.W.'s ophthalmic work during World War I in treating injured servicemen for free.

- Correspondence relating to the Oxford Ophthalmological Conference, July 1937.

- The D.J. Wood Memorial Lecture by Prof. J. L. van Selm, 1977.

- Tape recording of Donald Wood in conversation with Janet Hodgson (niece), recorded at Beachlands, Auckland, New Zealand, 12 November 2001.

♦ Tape Recording of Harry and Norah Wood in conversation with Janet Hodgson (daughter), recorded in Somerset West, 27 December 1990; and Harry's reminiscences recorded for his 90th birthday celebration, 24 January 1995. (He died on 4 February 1995).

♦ Geoffrey Montgomery (eldest living grandchild of David and Constance Wood, 80 in 2009), and Anne Montgomery: email correspondence with Janet Hodgson, 9 and 11April 2009.

(Some of this material is now deposited in the Department of Ophthalmology at Groote Schuur Hospital for archival purposes.)

✧

Bibliography

Bickford-Smith, Vivian, Elizabeth van Heyningen, Nigel Worden, *Cape Town in the Twentieth Century*, Cape Town: David Philip, 1999.

Bean, Lucy and Elizabeth van Heyningen, (eds.), *The Letters of Jane Elizabeth Waterston, 1866-1905*, Cape Town: The Van Riebeeck Society, 1983.

Benjamin, Harry, *Better Sight Without Glasses*, London: Health For All Publishing Co., 1929 (28th impression, 1952).

Berman, Esme, *Art and Artists of South Africa*, Cape Town: A.A. Balkema, 1983.

Blaxall, A.W., *Ten Cameos from Darkest Africa. Stories of Pioneer Work Amongst Coloured and African Blind*, Lovedale: Lovedale Press, 1937.

Burrows, Edmund H., *A History of Medicine in South Africa*, Cape Town: A.A. Balkema, 1958.

Daniell, G.W.B., ''The Mineral Waters of Caledon', Paper read at the Cape Town Medical Congress, 1893, *SAMJ*, 23 November 1940, pp.440-442.

Darley-Hartley, W., 'The Mineral Waters of Caledon', Paper read at the East London Medical Congress, 1908, *SAMJ*, 23 November, 1940, pp.437-440.

Davenport, T.R.H., *South Africa. A Modern History*, 2nd ed. Johannesburg: Macmillan South Africa, 1978.

Deacon, Harriet, 'The Medical Institutions on Robben Island' in Harriet Deacon (ed.), *The Island. A History of Robben Island, 1488-1990*, Cape Town and University of the Western Cape: David Philip and Mayibuye Books, 1996, pp.57-75.

De Villiers, J.C. (Kay) – oral history and D.J. Wood material in the Cape Medical Museum, May 2009.

De Villiers, J.C. (Kay), *Healers, Helpers and Hospitals. A History of Military Medicine in the Anglo-Boer War*, 3 Volumes, Pretoria: Protea Book House, 2009.

Du Plessis, G. 'The Life and Times of Dr DJ Wood - Part 1', 28th DJ Wood Memorial Lecture, February 2010, *SA Ophthalmology Journal*, 8 (2), Autumn 2013, pp.20-28.

Du Toit, J.S., 'In Memorium', *SAMJ*, August 1958, p.512.

Gibson, A.L.S., *Sketches of Church Work and Life in the Diocese of Capetown*, Cape Town: S.A. Electric Printing and Publishing, 1900.

Green, Lawrence G., *Secrets of Africa*, London: Stanley Paul, 1938; reprinted 1980, Cape Town: Howard Timmins.

♦ *So Few Are Free*, Cape Town: Howard Timmins, 1946.

♦ *Taverns of the Seas*, Cape Town: Howard Timmins, 1947.

♦ *In The Land Of Afternoon*, Cape Town: Howard Timmins, 1949.

- *Grow Lovely, Growing Old*, Cape Town: Howard Timmins, 1951.

- *A Decent Fellow Doesn't Work*, Cape Town: Howard Timmins, 1963.

- *I Heard The Old Men Say*, Cape Town: Howard Timmins, 1964.

Gutsche, Thelma, *No Ordinary Woman. The Life and Times of Florence Phillips*, Cape Town: Howard Timmins, 1966.

Herbert Baker biographical notes: www.sahistory.org.za.

Hutton, Barbara, *Robben Island. Symbol of Resistance*, Johannesburg and Cape Town: SACHED and Mayibuye Books, 1994.

Iacobuzio-Donahue, C. and N. Baker, *Hidden Beauty: Exploring the Aesthetics of Medical Science.* Atglen, Lancaster, Pennsylvania: Schiffer Publications, 2013.

Kannemeyer, J.C., 'Pediater, Pedagoog en Die Mediese Vereneging', in *Leipoldt, 'n Lewensverhaal*, Cape Town: Tafelberg, 1999.

Kerkham, Andrew Summers (ed.), 'Reminscences of William Andrew Kerkham, 2005, http://freepages.genealogy.rootsweb.ancestry.com/-kerkham/wak.htm: (originally published as *Forgotten times: Cape Town in the early twentieth century*, Cape Town: Friends of the South African Public Library, 1990).

Loos, Jackie, 'Light in a dark corner of apartheid', *Cape Argus*, December 13, 2000, p.17.

Louw, J.H., *In the Shadow of Table Mountain. A history of the University of Cape Town Medical School and its associated teaching hospitals up to 1950, with glimpses into the future*, Cape Town: Struik Publishing, 1969.

Louw, J.H. 'Leipoldt the paediatrician', *Suid-Afrikaanse Mediese Tydskrif (SAMJ)*, 6 December 1980.

Murray, A.D.N. 'Survival with Excellence: Ophthalmology today and in the Future', Inaugural Lecture as Helen and Morris Mauerberger Professor of Ophthalmology, University of Cape Town, New Series no.122, 3 September 1986.

Nel, G.D., *Jerseys in Southern Africa*, Cape Town: Tafelberg, 1968.

Newman, George, *Prize Essays in Leprosy*, London: The Society, 1895.

Penn, Nigel, Harriet Deacon, Neville Alexander, *Robben Island: The Politics of Rock and Sand*, University of Cape Town, 1992.

Pyzer, I., 'The Effects of Blue Light on Vision', email at info@medi-view.co.uk.

Retiina South Africa, *Information about Macular Degeneration*, sponsored by NOVARTIS.

Robinson, Helen, *Beyond the City Limits. People and Property at Wynberg, 1795-1927*, Cape Town: Juta & Co., 1998.

Robinson, Helen, *Wynberg. A Special Place*, Wynberg: Haughton House, 2001.

Rosenthal, E., *Fish Horns and Hansom Cabs. Life in Victorian Cape Town*, Cape Town: Ad Donker, 1977.

Rowland, W.P., *Being-Blind-in-the-World.* A Phenomenological Analysis of Blindness and a Formulation of New Objectives for Rehabilitation, Pretoria: National Council for the Blind, 1986.

Rowland, W. P., *Not About Us Without Us,* Pretoria: UNISA, 2004.

Staz, L., '*Random Reminiscences in the 40 Years lifetime of the Ophthalmological Society of South Africa*', published by OSSA, Johannesburg, n.d., pp.43-44.

Stuart-Findlay, D., 'The Siddeley Cup - Admission to the Sanatorium', *The Crankhandle Chronicle*, June 2013, pp.10-11.

Townsend, R.L.H., 'The Development of Ophthalmology in Cape Town', unpublished MS filed in the Ophthalmology Department, UCT, March 1962, 9 pages.

Van der Bijl, Pieter, 'Medical Art – a brief general overview, and its development in South Africa', student paper in *SAMJFoRUM, SAMJ*, 91 (12), December 2001.

Van Selm, J.L., 'Children with Learning Disabilities', the D.J. Wood Memorial Lecture, April 1979 – *Suid-Afrikaanse Argief vir Optalmologie*, 6 (1-4), Januarie-Desember 1979, pp.87ff.

Van Selm, J.L., 'Obituary: R.L.H. Townsend', filed in Ophthalmology Department, UCT.

Women of South Africa, 1913, Cape Town: Scribes Publishing.

✧

Appendix 1: The Children of David James and Constance Clara Wood

1. Howard James Faulkner. Born in Cape Town in 1897. Died in Pretoria, 1961. Doctor to the leper colony on Robben Island, until it was closed in the 1930s; then Deputy Superintendent to Westfort Leper Institute, Pretoria. Married to Triphena Fielding, a nurse. No children.

2. Marjorie (Madge) Constance Christina. Born in Cape Town on 1 September 1899. Died in Fish Hoek on 5 December, 1980. Married Alec (Rex) Marion Mayne Montgomery on 5 August 1925. They had 2 sons, David and Geoffrey, both born in Australia.

3. Harry Lawrence David. Born in Cape Town on 24 January 1904. Jersey cattle breeder and exporter of indigenous flora. Died in Somerset West on 4 February 1995. Married Norah Mary Janet Hill on 18 April 1931. They had 3 children, a daughter, Gillian and twins, James and Janet. Norah died in Somerset West on 30 March 1994.

4. Patricia (Patsy) Paula Landell. Born in Plumstead in 1907. First married Marshall Douglas-Jones. Divorced. Second marriage to Nobby Hall, who died in 1968. Third marriage to M.A. Garnett in Zimbabwe, who died in 1978.

Patsy had two daughters by her first husband, Nicolette and Veronica. She died in Australia in 1986.

5. Rosamund Griswold. Born in Plumstead on 27 August 1909. Married Neville Frederick Clayton, photographer, on 19 March 1934. Divorced. They had one son, John.

Second marriage to Edward Potter in 1943, and they had one son, Timothy. She died in 1974 in Pinetown, Natal.

6. Donald Nettleship Walker. Born in Plumstead in March 1912. Married Dorothy Heather-Noon, a highly qualified nursing sister, in 1943. They had 2 daughters and 2 sons, Heather and Barbara, Christopher and Michael. He died in New Zealand on 6 October 2006.

Appendix 2: Ophthalmic Notes, Addresses and Articles in South Africa by Dr. D.J.Wood

March 1894: Ophthalmic Notes: 'The Use of Eserine in Corneal Disease', *SAMJ*, I, p.226.

April 1894: Ophthalmic Notes: 'The Glands of the Ciliary Body', *SAMJ*, I, p.246.

May 1894: Ophthalamic Notes: 'Fluorescein', and 'Errors of Refraction and Epilepsy', *SAMJ*, II, pp.22-3.

June 1894: Ophthalmic Notes: 'Blinding of the Retina from Direct Sunlight', *SAMJ*, II, p.57.

July 1894: Ophthalmic Notes: 'Infective Ulceration of the Cornea', *SAMJ*, II, pp.73-4.

May 1895: Ophthalmic Notes: Miscellaneous Reports from other countries compared with local experience, *SAMJ*, III, pp.18-19.

July 1895: 'A Case of Hereditary Specific Iritis in a Young Child', read before the Cape Town Branch of the B.M.A, SAMJ, III, part 2, p.68.

July 1896: 'Two Cases of Diseases of the Eye. Patients shown before the Cape Town Branch of the B.M.A. Ciliary Staphyloma and Opthelmia Neonatorium', *SAMJ*, IV, part 3, p.63.

June 1903: Correspondence – Dr. Wood and the District Surgeons' Association, *SAMR*.

April 10, 1906: 'The Treatment of Bacterial Diseases by Vaccines', An

Inaugural Presidential Address to the C.G.H. (Western) Branch of the B.M.A., *SAMJ*, IV (6), pp.85-91.

June 28 1913: 'The Eye Complications of Leprosy', *SAMR*, XI, pp.245-6.

June 27, 1914: 'Oral and Intestinal Sepsis in Relation to the Diseases of Ophthalmic Patients', read at a combined meeting of C.G.H. (Western) Branch of B.M.A., and Dental Society of the Cape Province, *SAMR*, XII, pp.192-4.

October 28, 1922: 'Injuries and Common Diseases of the Eye', Introduction to a Discussion at the S.A. Medical Congress, 1922, *SAMJ*, XX, pp.390-8.

June 13, 1925: 'The Co-ordimeter of Prof. Ness', read before the Cape of Good Hope (C.G.H.) Branch of B.M.A, *SAMR*, XXIII, pp.235-6.

October 10, 1925: 'Some Cases of Retinal Disease Associated with Streptococcic Infection', read at 20th S.A. Medical Congress, *SAMR*, XXIII, pp.431-5.

November 14, 1925: 'The Optic Nerve Aspect of the Diagnosis of Intra-cranial Tumours', contribution to a Symposium at the Western Branch, B.M.A., *SAMR*, XXIII, pp.475-8.

October 13, 1928: 'Detachment of the Retina', *JMASA (B.M.A.)*, II, pp. 513-7.

January 10, 1931: 'An Ophthalmogical Society', Leading Article, *JMASA*, V (1).

January 10, 1931: Letter re 'An Ophthalmological Society', *JMASA*, V (1), p.29, and a further letter, V (2), p.30.

April 25, 1931: 'The Resistance of the Lamina Cribrosa as a Factor in Glaucoma' with two Scotoma Chart diagrams, *JMASA*, V (8), pp.251-4.

December 26, 1931: Inaugural Address at the first meeting of the Ophthalmological Society (September 1931), *JMASA,* V (24), pp.816-7.

December 26, 1931: 'Some Fundus Conditions', *JMASA,* V (24), pp.817-8.

March 1935: 'Staining of the Cornea by Blood-pigment', with a photograph of the general appearance of the eye earlier, and a drawing showing ruptures of iris on each side and above, *JMASA,* IX (5), pp.2-4.

November 1935: 'The Blindness of John Milton'. Monograph reprinted from *SAMJ.*

August 22, 1936: 'A Case of Supra-sellar Meningioma' with a photograph and eight Scotoma Chart diagrams, *SAMJ,* X (16), pp.580-3.

September 12, 1936: 'Clinical Notes. Avulsion of an Eye', *SAMJ,* X (17), p.611.

September 26, 1936: 'Trachoma Problems', *SAMJ,* X (17), pp. 629-31.

April 10, 1937: Announcement of the Death of Dr. D.J. Wood on Leader page, *SAMJ,* XI (7).

Appendix 3: Papers in the *British Journal of Ophthalmology* by D.J.Wood, Cape Town

September 1920: 'Three Cases of Total Removal of Iris', IV (9), pp.412-3.

September 1920: 'Detached Retina', IV (9), pp.413-5.

September 1920: 'Accommodative Failure in Malaria and Influenza', IV (9), pp.415-6.

March 1921: 'Conjunctival Pemphigus' with photograph, V (3), pp.121-4.

October 1922: 'Onyx of Long Duration' with drawing, VI (10), p.458.

October 1922: 'Intra-Ocular Cysticerus' with 2 small paintings of eyes, VI (10), pp.459-461.

January 1925: 'Ocular Leprosy', with 2 paintings, VIII (1), pp.1-4.

January 1925: 'Hyatid Cysts of the Orbit', VIII, pp.4-6.

September 1925: 'Two Cases of Non-Traumatic Cysts of the Anterior Chamber' with 2 paintings of Cysts by D.J.W. and 1 photograph, IX (9), pp.450-4.

May 1927: 'A Case of Sympathetic Ophthalmitis' with 6 photographs of sections on glass plates, XI (5), pp.217-24.

May 1927: 'Calcium Deficiency in the Blood with Reference to Spring Catarrh and Malignant Myopia', XI (5), pp.224-30.

August 1927: Letter – 'Calcium Deficiencies', XI (8), p.415.

March 1928: 'Melanosis of the Iris and New Formation of a Hyaline Membrane on its Surface' with a painting of a Slit-Lamp section, 4 photographs of bleached sections, and 4 photographs of unbleached sections on glass plates, XII (3), pp.140-3, together with 'Remarks' by E. Treacher Collins, pp.143-6.

June 1930: 'Two Cases of Sympathetic Ophthalmitis' with 12 photographs of sections on glass plates, XIV (6), pp.291-7.

July 1932: 'A Suggestion as to the Cause of Glaucoma Following Thrombosis of the Retinal Vein', XVI (7), pp.423-4.

September 1932: 'An Unusual Result Following Traumatic Irido-Cyclitis' with 3 photographs of sections on glass plates, XVI (9), pp.546-8.

March 1933: 'A Case of Congenital Cataract Showing Unusual Features'
with 2 paintings, of the left and right eyes, XVII (3), pp.158-61.

July 1935: 'Observations on the Human Retina' with 8 photographs of sections on glass plates, XIX (7), pp.369-377.

September 1936: 'Inflammatory Disease in the Eye Caused by Gout' with 7 large photographs of sections on glass plates, XX (9), pp.510-9.

June 1937: 'Obituary', XXI, pp.332-3.

July 17 1937: 'Night Blindness in Eye Diseases – Some Suggestions and Speculations', Doyne Memorial Lecture 1937, Report on the Oxford Ophthalmological Congress, *The British Medical Journal*, 17 July 1937, p.132.

Appendix 4: The D.J.Wood Memorial Lectures

1976 - Dr. Sam Etzine

1977 – Prof. Hennie Meyer

1978 – Prof. Neville Welsh

1979 – Prof. Justin van Selm: 'Children with Learning Disabilities'

1980 – Dr. E.T. Meyer

1985 – Dr. Geoff Howes

1986 – Dr. Hubrecht Brody: 'Ophthalmology: The Queen of Specialities – the Early Years'

1987 – Dr. Gavin Douglas

1989 – Dr. Francois Potgieter: 'Vitreoretinal Disorders in Perspective'

1990 – Prof. Basson van Rooyen: 'Pharmacokinetcs'

1991 – Dr. Selig Saks

1992 – Dr. John Bristow

1993 – Prof. Andries Stulting: 'The History of the Ophthalmological Society of South Africa: The Past, the Present and the Future'

1994 – Prof. Tony Murray: 'Does Strabismus Surgery Have a Functional Benefit?'

1995 – Dr. Werner Staples

1997 – Dr. John Hill: 'The Mechanism and Management of Corneal Graft Rejection'

1998 – Dr. John Venter

1999 – Prof. Anne Peters

2000 – Dr. Jan Talma

2001 – Dr. Colin Cook: 'Vision 20/20. The Right to Sight'

2002 – Dr. Johan A. de Lange

2004 – Dr. Ellen Ancker: 'Glaucoma'

2005 – Dr. Ivan Marais

2006 – Prof. Robert Stegmann: 'Remedies and Maladies in the Anterior Segment'

2007 – Dr. Elie Dahan: 'Doubts and Convictions in Ophthalmology'

2008 – Dr. Johann Slazus

2009 – Dr. Louis Kruger: 'Macular Holes'

2010 – Dr. G.P. du Plessis: 'The Life and Times of Dr. D.J. Wood (part 1), and Lessons Strabismus taught me (part 2)'

2011 – Dr. Asher Saks

2012 – Dr. Bill Nortje: 'Change in Ophthalmology'

2013 - Dr. Harold Konig: 'Professionalism'

Appendix 5: Paintings of the Retina by Tinus de Jongh and Dr. D.J.Wood in the Ophthalmological Department, Groote Schuur Hospital

Large signed original ochre paintings by Tinus De Jongh: Choroidal Tubercle:Thrombosis of the Retinal Vein. One unlabelled and unsigned.

Seminar Room – unsigned ochre paintings, all labelled Tinus de Jongh (copied by him from other works).

Central Choroiditis; Detachment of Retina; Albuminuric Retinitis Pregnancy Opaque Optic Nerve Fibres; Choroiditis; Disseminated Choroiditis; Normal Fundus

– Dark Type; Coloboma of Choroid; Central Choroiditis; Albumenuric Retinitis; Retinal Changes in Diabetes Choroiditis – probably tubercular; Retinitis circinata Retinitis proliferans.

Doctor's Passage D4 (different styles and mounted on different paper)

D.J. Wood – unsigned large ochre painting of Normal Fundus

D.J. Wood – unsigned large ochre painting of Detachment of Retina

D.J. Wood – unsigned large ochre painting of Pigmentary Retinitis

D.J. Wood signed – large ochre painting of Papilloedema

De Jongh – unsigned ochre painting of Optic Atrophy

De Jongh – unsigned ochre painting of Early Papilloedema

The Library – unsigned ochre paintings labelled Tinus de Jongh: Early Disseminated Choroiditis; Albumenuric Retinitis Pregnancy; Ruptures of the Choroid Embolism of Retinal Artery; Myopic Degeneration; Disseminated Choroiditis – Late Stage.

The Library – Dr. Wood's paintings – signed and unsigned

Raised sub retinal exudate. H.P. Left eye (signed)

Sister Magdalene, January – May 1930 (unsigned)

Gumma of Iris 1924

Blasting accident. Fragments of stone in the Iris (signed) + Vitreous prolapse sub capsular cataract trauma in the same frame (unsigned)

Extensive raised subretinal exudate. 1929. Rt. Eye. Peterson (signed)

Modular scleritis

Melanoma of Iris

Retinal Amacroma (now called aneurism)

Leprotic Iritis (signed) and Leprotic infiltration of Cornea - pubished in *BJO*, January 1925, VIII, pp.1-4.

Cyst of Anterior Chamber. F55. OC.2 – published in *BJO*, September 1925, IX, pp.450-4.

Cataracts – published in *BJO*, XVII, March 1932, pp.158-161.

Also mounted photographs of 2 histology slides – 2 Iris Cysts endothelial cells on surface X 400

The library also has a small museum (2 glass cases) of ophthalmic interest, curated by Professor Tony Murray. He has included a photo of an operation for Cataract

146

surgery (patient seated) – Karl Himly (1772-1837); and a series of photos giving the different stages in a cataract operation, 1957.

The Outpatient Department has a small museum curated by Professors Tony Murray and Colin Cook. This includes a museum case with 9 wooden trays with 8 glass jars in each of Dr. Wood's pathological specimens, all labelled. In a glass-fronted cupboard are 3 of his boxes of photographic plates of clinical cases and pathology specimens. About 10cm square in size, the details of each plate are listed on the box lids. There are also a number of photographs on glass plates, some published in the *BJO*. One longer box contains images on glass plates to use with children, imported from England, e.g. camels, frogs, spiders, spider webs, dove cot and bird, horse, mouse, little men, house, clock, swing, flags, large and small squares, large and small red dots, green stripes, etc.

Acknowledgements

I am indebted to many people who have encouraged and supported me in writing this book, especially my four children and their spouses – Michael and Julie, James and Arlene, Alastair and Tracy, Carol and Tim – and my six grandsons. My daughter-in-law, Julie, has become our family historian and has devoted many hours to doing research on the Wood family tree, and filing all available records. This included assisting in the collection of D.J.Wood's articles in South African and British medical journals held in the Groote Schuur Hospital library. Julie has also been responsible for assembling the Wood family photographs, and taking the pictures of both Tinus de Jongh's and D.J.W.'s drawings and paintings at Groote Schuur, as well as D.J.W.'s material in the Medical Museum in Cape Town. She has now put these all together on a CD.

My eldest son, Mike, was also drawn in when I raided his complete collection of Lawrence G. Green's books; while my daughter, Carol, has done research and typing for me and provides invaluable back up. My grandson, Gareth Hodgson, was even hijacked into putting a power point presentation together with skills quite beyond my competency. The recollections of my cousin, Geoff Montgomery, have added much to the family's history and we are all greatly indebted to him for his contribution.

I need to express my gratitude, too, to faithful friends and neighbours in McGregor and Somerset West, who have shared my joys and tribulations, and provided me with so much support. Lyle Jobling, a near neighbour, has helped me to track down the historica paintings at Groote Schuur Hospital, did some last minute proofreeading and continues to offer assistance in many different ways, including driving me around. Dr. Ann Haw is another who has given me invaluable help.

I am grateful to Dr. Leonard Townsend for all he did for me as a child. In recent years, Dr. Stephan van Dijk of Worcester, and Dr. Gavin Bingham of Somerset West, have done what they could to preserve and improve my vision. Elspeth Campbell and Bev Richardson of the Helen Keller Society in Pinelands, provide ongoing advice in their monthly meetings of the Low Vision Support Group in Somerset West. Thanks to their visual aids I have been able to continue writing. I follow their 3 Bs mantra for Low Vision – Bigger, Brighter, Bolder. These really work.

As medical historians, Professor 'Kay' de Villiers, former Head of Neurosurgery, and Professor Anthony (Tony) Murray, former Head of Ophthalomology at UCT, inspired me to get going on this biography in 2009; but I was then waylaid by other writing. More recently new friends have provided invaluable help. Derek Stuart-Findley in Cape Town, an authority on classic cars, researched the Automobile Association magazines to come up with original material and exact dates of D.J.W.'s motoring exploits. Jackie Loos, journalist and librarian, assisted in tracing material relating to the Athlone School for the Blind. Richard Keeler, Hon. Curator of the Royal College of Ophthalmologists and Hon. Archivist of the Moorfields Alumni Association, sent me old photographs from the Eye Hospital.

Professor Colin Cook and Professor Anthony Murray traced the fundus (retina) paintings and drawings done by my grandfather and Tinus de Jongh, now framed and hanging in various sections of the Ophthalmological Department at Groote Schuur Hospital. More recent foraging in the hospital's storage department has uncovered yet more exciting finds. Professor Cook has mounted a display of D.J.W.'s pathological specimens in their glass jars, as well as four boxes of photographic glass plates of clinical cases and pathology specimens, all labelled. These are now exhibited in their small museum in the Outpatient Department. Professor Murray's detective work came up with more watercolour paintings of eyes, most signed D.J.W. I am immensely grateful to Professor Cook for allowing me to make numerous trips to his department to photograph these finds and for graciously putting up with my badgering to obtain all the necessary information. All the photos have been recorded on a CD as archival material in addition to a selection for this book.

In Manchester, the Revd. Jayant Kothare has assisted with research and has spent many long hours in proofreading and editing the manuscript, usually at short notice. I would never have been able to finish this task without his long-distant support and helpful advice on many aspects of the story. We have now worked together for twenty-seven years on many of my publications, and he has been a tower of strength throughout.

I am particularly grateful to Dr. Gideon du Plessis for sending me the information he had on my grandfather, some of which he personally researched in the U.K. This formed Part 1 of his D.J.Wood Memorial Lecture in 2010 and was received with great interest. He has a large collection of photos, too. Dr. du Plessis has read through this manuscript and has given ongoing support and advice, which I have greatly valued. I am indebted to him for doing the Foreword, too, in the midst of a busy practice, and for all he has to say about my grandfather's work and contributions, which are heartfelt in their integrity. Unfortunately, no record has been kept of the topics for the D.J.Wood Memorial Lectures since 1976, but Professor Andries Stulting and Dr. Hubrecht Brody have done all they could to fill in the gaps. The list is still incomplete.

Dr. William Rowland, Past President of the World Blind Unit and Honorary Life President of both the S.A. National Council for the Blind and Disabled People South Africa (amongst many other honours), has opened new doors in my research. Blinded in a shooting incident at the age of four, he has been an inspiration as a writer and poet, and advocate for the disabled. I hope that renewed interest in my grandfather will contribute towards the funding of his Audio Describe project for blind and visually impaired people. This cause has become very important to me as with my own failing eyesight I realise how such a project could enrich the lives of those so disabled. To crown it all he has added an Epilogue, which contributes an important dimension to the different perspectives given on D.J.W.'s life and work. In reading the manuscript his encyclopaedic memory saved me from making a number of errors

Lastly, I must thank Derek Thomas who has done the design and layout of the book, organised the printing, and managed the electronic processing. Much of this is beyond my comprehension but he has been marvellously efficient and endlessly patient. I am delighted with the results.

✦

Publications by Janet Hodgson

Ntsikana's Great Hymn: a Xhosa Expression of Christianity in the 19ᵗʰ Century Eastern Cape. UCT: Centre for African Studies, 1980.

The God of the Xhosa. Cape Town:OUP, 1982.

Princess Emma. Johannesburg: Ad Donker, 1987.

Vision Quest. Native Spiritualityand the Church in Canada, co-authored with the Revd. Jayant Kothare. Toronto: Anglican Book Centre, 1990.

The Faith We See. Working with Images of Christ (with CD Rom). Peterborough: Inspire, Methodist Publishing House, 2006.

Making the Sign of the Cross (Creative Resources for seasonal worship, retreats and quiet days – a work book with CD Rom). London and Norwich: SCM-Canterbury Press, 2010.

Seeing Our Faith. (Creative ideas for working with Images of Christ – a work book with CD Rom). London and Norwich: SCM-Canterbury Press, 2011.

Good News Story Workshops (based on the 5 Marks of Mission). Cambridge: Grove Books, EV 95, 2011.

Living With Low Vision. Cape Town, 2014.

List of photographs: Julie Hodgson

1. David James Wood   - Cover Picture (by Neville Clayton, son-in-law)
2. David James Wood's Birth Certificate
3. Wood Family, Earlston – James and Christina with David James and Harriet
4. Moorfields Eye Hospital, London, near Finsbury Circus, 1875
5. 'View of the Human Eye', from Harry Benjamin, *Better Sight Without Glasses,* London: Health For All Publishing Company, first published 1929
6. Prescription, dated 12.I.1925, signed D.J.W. (in the possession of Professor Andries Stulting)
7. 'Gledsmuir' from the vlei, with Table Mountain in the background, photograph taken by D.J.W. in the early 1910s. Murray Bisset's house is on the left
8. 'Gledsmuir', Southfield Road, Plumstead
9. D.J.W. as winner of the Siddeley Cup trial, 1912, with September, the chauffeur, up front and family in the back seat
10. Line up of cars for the Siddeley Cup trial, 1912, D.J.W. to the extreme left
11. Caledon Baths Sanatorium Hotel and Baths – advertisement
12. D.J. Wood in one of his cars with a young daughter
13. D.J.W.'s wooden trays with 8 jars of pathological specimens in each, Ophthalmology Department Museum, Groote Schuur Hospital
14. Label on pathogenic specimen of 'Mrs. Brown, 1920, Wound by stick. Cornea adhered to remains of Lens…Excised for pain', Ophthalmology Museum, Groote Schuur Hospital

15. Tinus de Jongh
16. Unsigned painting by Tinus de Jongh of 'Retinitis Proliferans' (c.1923-4), Seminar Room, Ophthalmology Department, Groote Schuur Hospital
17. Unsigned painting by Tinus de Jongh of 'Albumenuric Retinitis Pregnanacy' (c.1923-4), Seminar Room, Ophthalmology Department, Groote Schuur Hospital
18. Signed fundus painting by Tinus de Jongh, Ophthalmology Department, Groote Schuur Hospital (c.1923-4)
19. Constance Clara Wood at 'Gledsmuir'
20. Dr. David James and Constance Clara Wood with Patsy and Rosamund (youngest daughters)
21. Constance Clara Wood at 'Gledsmuir'
22. Harry Wood, D.J.W.'s second son and Janet Hodgson's father
23. Harry Wood's prize-winning Jersey cows, Rosebank Show, 1952
24. Slit-lamp painting by D.J.W. of 'Melanosis of the Iris and New Formation of a Hyaline Membrane on its Surface', *BJO (XII)*, March 1928.
25. Slit-lamp painting (X15 diameter) of 'Leprotic Iritis' by D.J.W. in 'Ocular Leprosy', *BJO (VIII)*, January 1925
26. Two signed D.J.W. watercolour paintings, 1925. At the top - 'Blasting accident. Fragments of Stone in the Iris'. Below – 'Vitreous Prolapse Subcapsular Cataract Trauma', Ophthalmology Department Library, Groote Schuur Hospital
27. Photographic Glass Plate of a Dovecote and three birds.
28. Photographic Glass Plate of a Camel, Ophthalmology Department Museum, Groote Schuur Hospital
29. Four boxes of D.J.W.'s Photographic Glass Plates, Ophthalmology Department Museum, Groote Schuur Hospital
30. D.J.W.'s Phials with specimens removed from eyes mounted on a wooden board with explanatory notes typed underneath, Ophthalmology Department Museum, Groote Schuur Hospital
31. Signed watercolour painting by D.J.W., 'Extensive Raised Subretinal Exudate++WR H.P. 1929 Rt, Eye, Ophthalmology Department, Groote Schuur Hospital
32. Signed painting by D.J.W. of 'Papilloedema', Doctors' Passage, Ophthalmology Department, Groote Schuur Hospital
33. Dr. F.C. Louis Leipoldt
34. Signed watercolour painting by D.J.W. of 'Raised sub retinal exudate. H.P. Left Eye', Ophthalmology Department Library, Groote Schuur Hospital
35. D.J.W. painting – Retinal Amacroma (now called aneurism), Ophthalmology Department Museum, Groote Schuur Hospital
36. Dr. David James Wood
37. Dr. Janet Hodgson (photograph by Cornel Hough).

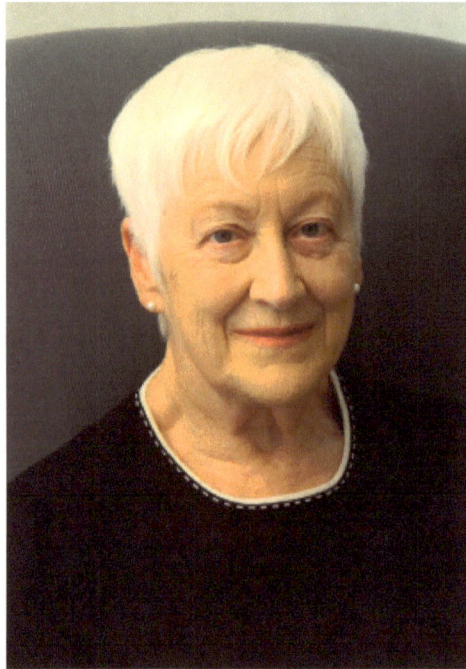

Dr. Janet Hodgson
(photograph by Cornel Hough) (37)

www.ingramcontent.com/pod-product-compliance
Lightning Source LLC
Chambersburg PA
CBHW041454210326
41599CB00005B/244